THE RUNNER'S HANDBOOK TRAINING DIARY

Bob Glover, a sub-three-hour marathoner and competitive runner for fifteen years, has had a multifarious athletic career. In Vietnam in 1969 he organized and directed the "Hue Olympics," attracting thousands of visitors to a burned-out stadium that had once been headquarters for the North Vietnamese Army. As fitness director of New York City's West Side Y.M.C.A., he developed and led the country's largest fitness program, with over three thousand participants. He has run in twenty-six marathons, one fifty-kilometer race, and one fifty-miler on a track, as well as in the Mount Washington Race (eight miles up the Northeast's highest peak). He is also founder and coach of the Greater New York Athletic Association, whose women's team is now of national caliber. Recently, he founded Robert H. Glover and Associates, Inc., a physical-fitness consulting firm serving a variety of corporate and community clients.

Jack Shepherd was graduated from Haverford College and Columbia University but says, "I really got my education as a senior editor at Look magazine during the 1960s, when I covered the civil-rights movement, drugs, Berkeley, etc." As an author-journalist he has traveled in forty-six of the fifty United States and the Far East, Europe, the Caribbean, and Africa. Articles by him have appeared in Newsweek, Harper's, the Saturday Review, Reader's Digest, The New York Times Sunday Magazine, and other periodicals; he is the author or coauthor of seven previous books—among them The Forest Killers, nominated for a National Book Award, and his second bestseller, The Adams Chronicles. After a recent trip to East Africa he began Bob Glover's running program, which, he decided, deserved to be the subject of a book, The Runner's Handbook, which he coauthored with Mr. Glover and which became a national bestseller.

The Runner's Handbook Training Diary

Bob Glover and Jack Shepherd

Penguin Books

Penguin Books Ltd, Harmondsworth,
Middlesex, England
Penguin Books, 625 Madison Avenue,
New York, New York 10022, U.S.A.
Penguin Books Australia Ltd, Ringwood,
Victoria, Australia
Penguin Books Canada Limited, 2801 John Street,
Markham, Ontario, Canada L3R 1B4
Penguin Books (N.Z.) Ltd, 182–190 Wairau Road,
Auckland 10, New Zealand

First published 1978

LIBRARY OF CONGRESS CATALOGING IN PUBLICATION DATA
Glover, Bob.
   The runner's handbook training diary.
   1. Running–Training–Forms.   I.   Shepherd, Jack,
joint author.   II.   Title.
GV1061.5.G56   796.4'26   78-15263
ISBN 0 14 046.373 9

Printed in the United States of America by
Offset Paperback Mfrs., Inc., Dallas, Pennsylvania
Set in VIP Electra and Janson

Contents

The Runner's Handbook Training Diary

How to use this diary

This is a runner's training diary. You are the writer.

This diary is designed for every runner from beginner to competitor. In it you can enter your day-to-day training record (pages 42-146), your weekly and monthly mileage (pages 146-150), your best races and personal records (pages 152-153), your favorite running courses (page 151), and much more. The diary will help you keep a record of every aspect of your running life, from how you feel each day to how long you run, from your resting heart rate to the wear and tear on your running shoes.

The Runner's Handbook Training Diary contains training tips and historical notes, races and racing contacts, pace and weight charts, lists of publications, guidelines about diet, shoes, clothing, training, and other useful information. But at its heart is the runner's personal week-at-a-glance diary. Whatever your running level, the diary will help you keep an accurate record of your progress up the training ladder.

Why record your progress? The past is a valuable guide to the future. In the diary, you set goals and plan your training program. You describe in it what you did and how it felt. The diary contains the facts of your training and doesn't leave them to memory.

The diary, when filled in, also becomes a guide and reference. It is a record of your training. If you are a beginner, you will be able to see and measure your growth as a runner. If you are training for your first race, or your next marathon, the diary will help you train regularly and train well. It will contain an accurate daily account of your workouts. Afterward, you will be able to look back to your training schedule to see what you did right (or wrong) in preparing for a race (or reaching a fitness level). You can then repeat this training procedure (or see your progress) or avoid past mistakes. The goals you set and your training to reach them become results you can review in the *Training Diary* in the future.

Be consistent in keeping your diary. Fill it in each day after your workouts.

In the week-at-a-glance, record the details of your runs: the conditions, whom you ran with, your weight and pulse, the weather, pace, distance, your health, feelings—even the personal things unrelated to running, like birthdays or first encounters with new friends.

Pages 36-39 contain two sample week-at-a-glance diaries. The first illustrates how a beginner runner, in this case a woman, might use the diary during a typical week early in her training program. The second sample illustrates how a competitor, here a man, might record entries in his training diary.

Several features should be noted. Both runners, although at different levels, use the Shoes entry. The woman keeps a record of her new running shoes. The man has numbered his several pairs of running shoes and records the mileage on each and how they feel and wear.

Both runners also record either distance or time in the designated box—but not distance *and* time.

Notice, too, that both runners take days off, and both walk and run on days when they don't feel in top form. Both record resting heart rates and weight. The beginner will soon be able to look back and see each condition decrease.

For both runners, the training diary is a record not just of their running but also of their health. Make the diary your recording tool for getting fit and staying fit. It may become the most important book of your life.

Step one: Seek medical advice

Anyone who is beginning to run—whether or not you consider yourself a beginner—should get a medical check-up. Any strenuous exercise program should be approved by your physician.

If you are over thirty-five, or under thirty-five and your medical history includes one major risk factor (smoking more than a pack of cigarettes a day, hypertension, hyperlipidemia, obesity, diabetes), your physical examination should include blood tests and a stress electrocardiogram.

Runners who decide to increase their mileage to train for a marathon are also advised to first consult their runner-doctor.

Any runner who develops a running-related illness or injury that interferes with his or her training should seek advice from a sports medicine expert.

Beware of nonexercising doctors. If your doctor doesn't run, invite him or her along for your next workout.

The run-easy method

All runners run easy, run long, run aerobically.

All runners use three basic training steps: Warm-up, Run, Cool-down. For most, only the time or distance of the run varies.

Warm-up. Before running, take 15 minutes to perform some relaxation, flexibility, and stretching exercises. A muscle works best when it is at maximum length. This involves slow, rhythmic stretching, stopping and holding at the point of first discomfort. Hold your stretch for 15-30 seconds. Never jerk or bounce in stretching. These exercises can also be done on your rest days.

There are some 15 basic stretching and relaxation exercises detailed for this program, plus about 100 supplemental exercises, in *The Runner's Handbook*. For example, the Sitting Stretch: Sit up, legs apart, hands together, and arms outstretched. Slide the fingers down one leg as far as possible, and hold. Keep the back of your knee flat against the ground. If you can reach your toes, pull them gently. Hold and return to sitting position. Repeat on other leg. Do three sets. Then put feet together, slide hands down legs as far as you can, and hold. Do not jerk or force the stretch.

Both abdominal and upper body strength is important for runners. This does not mean becoming musclebound, but developing the muscles along the front of your body to compensate for muscles along your back, hamstrings and calves, strengthened by running. For minimal development of abdominal and upper body muscles, sit-ups and push-ups should be performed during the warm-up. Sit-ups should be performed with your knees bent. (See pages 32-33 of *The Runner's Handbook*.) Weight training is also of benefit (see pages 15-16, 121-123 of the *Handbook*).

The run. This is the core of the Run-Easy Method. Beginners will run and walk; the key is to walk until you are ready to run, run until you want to walk. Also, run at a pace that enables you to talk with a companion or to hum. (See page 15 of this *Diary*.) Start your run by walking for at least 5 minutes.

All runners should run aerobically. This provides excellent training for your cardiovascular system. Your "target zone" of beneficial and safe training falls between two numbers: the target rate of 70 percent of your maximum heart rate, and the cut-off figure of 85 percent maximum heart rate (see table). The pulse rates are based upon a predicted maximum; they are only guides. Use the "talk test" to monitor your speed as a beginner runner.

The following table designates heart rates in various age groups (rates apply to both men and women).

Age	Target hr (70%)	Cut-off hr (85%)
20–25	140	167
26–30	134	163
31–35	131	159
36–40	127	155
41–45	124	150
46–50	120	146
51–55	117	142
56–60	113	138
61–65	110	133
66–70	106	129

Cool-down.   Walk after your run. Your heart rate should drop below 120; 110 if you are over fifty. If it doesn't, walk some more.

The Cool-down is the Warm-up in reverse. Repeat the stretching exercises, performing them slowly and rhythmically.

For a complete description of the Run-Easy Method, its exercises and diagrams, consult *The Runner's Handbook*, pages 29-66, 121-136, 341-346.

Minimum exercise chart

To achieve a minimum level of fitness, Dr. Kenneth Cooper recommends that you cover, in your chosen form of exercise, at least this mileage per week.

Bicycle: 30 miles per week
Walking: 15 miles per week
Swimming: 1.5 miles per week
Running: 6 miles per week

Three basic questions

1. HOW OFTEN SHOULD I RUN?

The beginner runner should run or run/walk at least three, four, or five times a week. The intermediate runner—who runs 30 consecutive minutes at a comfortable pace—and the beginner racer should run four to six days a week. The serious competitive runner runs daily, and sometimes twice a day.

Older runners will need more rest days, since their bodies take longer to recover after stressful running. All runners should not hesitate to take a day or more off to allow recovery from injury, illness, or staleness.

2. HOW FAST SHOULD I RUN?

Beginner and intermediate runners should do all their training at a slow, easy, and comfortable pace. "Train, don't strain." The speed should be at a conversational pace: if you can't talk comfortably and run at the same time, slow down or walk briskly and start again when you've caught your breath.

More serious runners should do 70 to 90 percent of their training at a conversational pace. They should add speed workouts, time trials, races, and so forth to their base work in order to develop the ability to run at an uncomfortable (anaerobic) but rewarding race pace.

3. HOW LONG SHOULD I RUN?

Beginners start by running, or running/walking, for at least 20 consecutive minutes. The next step, if you wish to go beyond the minimum standards, is gradually to extend the run to 30 to 60 minutes. In terms of distance, that would be running about a mile or two at first and extending to about three to six miles. Remember: run either for time or distance, but not both; that's racing.

Increase your distance from one week to the next by no more than 10 to 20 percent. Beware of sudden changes in your training.

Running style

Footstrike. Run the way you walk, heel to toe. Footstrike should not be toe first. You should gently land on the heel and gently roll forward to the ball of the foot and then push off. Your well-cushioned shoes are thick in the heel for a reason: to absorb the major impact of your weight as you run.

Stride. Don't over-stride. Your front foot should land almost directly under your front knee. Over-striding may cause knee and leg injury.

Style. Run erect but comfortably, with hands loosely cupped and arms carried low, between the waistline and chest. Some runners, to relax, form an "O" with each hand by touching thumb to middle finger. Others deliberately run with their hands and fingers open, to feel the wind. Hand stiffness and rigidity may tighten your shoulders and back.

Use your arms to move you along. Don't just carry them for the ride. Make the movement of your arms pull you along. Arms balance the runner; the left arm swings forward with the right leg, the right arm with the left leg. Use your arms to propel you uphill.

Breathing. Relax, and learn to belly-breathe. As you breathe in, your stomach should expand. This will help you to take in more oxygen and prevent side stitches.

Breathe in any way you can. Get all the air you need. Frank Shorter suggests an occasional long, deep breath released slowly that may help you relax. This is also good before a race.

Remember the Three R's of running: run tall, run relaxed, run naturally.

Your running program

You can start a running program any time. Of course, the sooner the better. This *Training Diary* will help you measure your progress, whether that is toward a minimal level of fitness, or a marathon.

Remember to have a medical check-up. As Joe Henderson says, "You can't be fit without first being healthy."

These programs are geared for five general levels: beginner runner, intermediate runner, beginner racer, beginner marathoner, competitive runner. Each of the levels overlaps somewhat. Runners may want to progress from beginner to marathoner or stop along the way when they reach a condition of fitness best for them. (Complete details of these programs are contained in *The Runner's Handbook*, pages 17-109.)

Each level also has its own training chart. All the charts are guides and set general running goals. You may follow them closely or adapt their information to your own running program. Whichever you do, be sure to record your training results in your week-at-a-glance diary.

Decide which level runner you are. Be sure you fit the criteria for that level. Be honest: you are only competing against the old, out-of-shape you. You don't want to risk injury. Perhaps you should start at an easier level and work up. Enter the results in your diary and watch your progress.

Select your level. Begin your training program any place on the chart that feels comfortable. For example, if you are a beginner and can meet the training requirements of Week Four, start there. Progress as fast as you wish. Remember: Take it easy. "Train, don't strain."

If you miss some running time because of injury or illness, back up a few weeks and start again. If you walk, also use the diary to record your walking.

Runners at every level should remember that it is all right, and even advisable, to walk as well as run.

Beginner runner

A beginner runner is someone who cannot jog comfortably for 20 consecutive minutes.

Here are some basic guidelines this runner should follow:

- Always stretch before and after your workouts. (The Warm-up and Cool-down phases of the Run-Easy Method.) This is essential to avoid injury.

The Run-Easy Method for beginner runners involves 20 minutes of continuous movement. At first, you walk before you run. You can probably walk for 20 to 30 minutes now. Your "run," therefore, may consist of 20 minutes of brisk walking. Gradually, you will replace the walking with running, until you can run for the entire 20 minute period. Listen to your body. If you want a structured program follow the chart on page 16.

Walk until you feel ready to run, and run until you need to walk again. Tip: Run comfortably at a conversational pace until you are short of breath—or your legs yell for rest—and then walk until you are ready to run again. Remember to run at a pace that enables you to talk with a companion or to hum if alone. This is the "talk test." If you are out of breath, slow down or walk.

- To build exercise benefits, walk or run at least three days a week, preferably four. Don't lay off more than two days in a row.
- No time? Make an appointment with yourself to run. Put that hour aside for yourself, and guard it.
- Take your pulse before, during, and after your runs. Follow the aerobic

heart rate chart on page 12. Your Cool-down pulse should be 100 or less; if not, keep walking. Record your pulse and weight in the diary.

- Wear good running shoes. Do not run in sneakers or similar shoes. Follow the tips on clothing, running style, shoes, diet in this *Training Diary* and *The Runner's Handbook*.
- Finally, be patient. The first few weeks are the toughest. Persist. Be consistent in your workouts. Note every inch of progress in your daily record.
- Smile! You're on the road to fitness.

Beginner runner's chart

How to use it. Begin with Week One, and progress slowly. Be sure to Warm-up and Cool-down. The Warm-up is followed by five minutes of progressively brisk walking, and then your run/walk. As a beginner, you will start by walking more than running for the 20-minute "run." That ratio slowly changes as you progress until you can run for 20 minutes.

For example, in Week One, you start with 15 minutes of stretching Warm-up, a 5-minute brisk walk, and then the 20-minute workout. You may walk the whole 20 minutes, or follow the chart, which suggests that

Beginner runner's eight-week program

| | Warm-up | | |
Week	Stretching (minutes)	Walk (minutes)	The run/walk
1	15	5	Run 1 minute, walk 2 minutes, six times. Run 1 more minute and walk 1. (Total: 20 minutes)
2	15	5	Run 1 minute, walk 1, ten times
3	15	5	Run 2 minutes, walk 1, six times. Run 2 more minutes at end
4	15	5	Run 3 minutes, walk 1 minute, five times
5	15	5	Run 4 minutes, walk 1, four times
6	15	5	Run 6 minutes, walk 1, twice, followed by a 6-minute run
7	15	5	Run 8 minutes, walk 1, twice, followed by a 2-minute run.
8	15	5	One 20-minute run

you run 1 minute, walk 2 minutes, and repeat this combination six times, followed by a 1-minute run and 1-minute walk (that makes 20 minutes). Next, walk 5 minutes and perform 10 minutes of Cool-down stretching exercises.

Remember that the chart is a guide. It may not be necessary for you to follow it closely, or you may want the structure it will give your running program. Progress at your own pace.

The goal is to reach 20 consecutive minutes of running. You begin each day by stretching, walking, then run/walk for 20 minutes, then walking and finally the Cool-down stretching. Each workout day, enter in the column marked "Actual" the number of minutes you ran, and compare it to the daily total to the left of that column. Enter in your diary your daily and weekly totals.

Beginner runners should run three to four days a week. A sample schedule might look like this:

Monday	Tuesday	Wednesday	Thursday	Friday	Saturday	Sunday
Off	20 min run/walk	Off	20 min run/walk	Off	20 min run/walk	Off or 20 min run/walk

Total daily run		Cool-down	
Goal (minutes of running)	Actual	Walk (minutes)	Stretching (minutes)
7		5	10
10		5	10
14		5	10
15		5	10
16		5	10
18		5	10
18		5	10
20		5	10

Intermediate runner

An intermediate runs 20 minutes a day, three to five times a week. He or she has reached a minimal level of fitness and may decide to stay there or to go on.

This is the transitional step in running. You are not a beginner, yet you are not ready to enter your first race. To build toward that goal, if you wish, follow these simple guidelines.

- Stay at your training schedule of 20 minutes, three to five days a week. Build this base for four weeks. Next, slowly increase your running to 30 minutes a day, five days a week. The following chart shows how. Tip: Never increase your weekly mileage by more than ten to 20 percent.
- Continue to spend 15 minutes in Warm-up stretching and 10 minutes in Cool-down. Remember to run at a conversational pace. Before you run, continue to jog slowly until you reach your workout pace, and afterwards as you lead into your Cool-down.

Intermediate runner's chart

How to use it. After building a four-week base beyond the beginner runner level, slowly increase your continuous running time according to the chart.

Week	Running time (minutes)	Days per week
1	22	three to five
2	25	three to five
3	27	four to five
4	30	five

SAMPLE WEEK

Monday	Tuesday	Wednesday	Thursday	Friday	Saturday	Sunday
Off	30 min	20-30 min	30 min	Off	20-30 min or Off	30 min

At this time, you may want to shift from thinking about running in terms of minutes to thinking about it in terms of miles (or kilometers). Most beginner and intermediate runners are in the 9- to 10-minute-per-mile category. At that speed, a 20-minute workout would cover about 2 miles; 30 minutes, about 3 miles or more.

You may also want to shift your thinking from fitness to racing.

Beginner racer

You are running 30 minutes a day, three to five days a week. Or you are running 3 miles a day, four days a week (12 miles a week). Believe it or not, you are ready for your first race.

Don't be put off. This is the era of the fun racer. The majority of racers today are in it for the enjoyment.

For your first race, pick a distance of between 3 and 6 miles (5 to 10 kilometers). Choose simple goals: to pin your number on correctly, to get the "feel" of competition, and to finish.

To finish any race comfortably, follow this basic rule. You should be running twice the race distance every week for four weeks before race day. Included in this should be two runs of two-thirds the race distance. For example, your first race might be 10 kilometers (6.2 miles). Four weeks before the race you should be running at least 12 miles a week, with two or more runs before the race of about 4 miles each. This basic level will enable you to finish the 10-kilometer run.

Better yet, cover three times the race distance for one month before the starting gun. Include at least two easy runs of race distance or more. Now you are ready to compete comfortably and will be able to raise your arms in a victory "V" as you cross the finish line. You will have won *your* race!

Here are some guidelines for the beginner racer.

- Remember the rule: Increase your mileage by only 10 to 20 percent per week.
- On your off days, perform flexibility exercises and walk.
- Run all training workouts at about your comfortable race pace goal.
- Don't bother to buy racing shoes yet. Also, don't race in new running shoes. Well-cushioned running shoes will minimize the chances for injury.
- Mark off your running course with a few mile markers. Note the landmarks and distances in your diary. On some training days, carry a stopwatch to measure your most comfortable running pace. Use the charts in the back of your diary (page 146). Most races have mileage markers for pacing purposes. You may also want to carry the stopwatch

during your first few races to condition yourself to your own race pace. Later, you'll know it well and run it easily.

On race day:

- Stretch before the race.
- Don't overdress or underdress (see Seasonal Tips, pages 32-35).
- Start slow, build your speed gradually. Walk if you need to, but keep moving.
- If it is hot, drink fluids before, during, and after the race.
- Carbohydrate-loading is for marathons, not for shorter races. Follow your normal diet during the week of the race. On race day, eat nothing, or something very light that agrees with you.
- Set a reasonable race goal: To finish comfortably.
  Recovery: Walk off the course and keep moving. Stretch. Take a warm bath. Gradually return to your training schedule. Plot strategy for your next race. (For help, see *The Runner's Handbook*, pages 86-91.)
- Be sure to keep a careful record of your training in this diary. You will want to refer to it for future races.

Beginner racer's training program for ten-

Week	Monday		Tuesday		Wednesday		Thursday	
	Goal	Actual	Goal (miles)	Actual (miles)	Goal (miles)	Actual (miles)	Goal (miles)	Actual (miles)
1	Off		2		3		3	
2	Off		3		3		3	
3	Off		3		4		3	
4	Off		3		4		4	
5	Off		3		4		3	
6	Off		2		4		3	
7	Off		4		3		3	
8	Off		4		3		2	

Beginner racer's chart

How to use it. This chart is a guide for the man or woman building up to a 10-kilometer race. The schedule is flexible. You can change the days and mileage, modify it to your own development, or follow the chart closely. Be sure to fill in your training times in the "Actual" column.

The chart assumes that your race is on a Sunday and allows an eight-week build up. Week Six is the key to your training.

Note the hard-easy method of training, plus the tapering off. This is the pattern followed for all races. Remember: Warm-up and Cool-down remain essential.

Remember to smile when you complete your race, and remember that in our sport every finisher has won his or her race!

---

kilometer race

Friday		Saturday		Sunday		TOTALS	
Goal (miles)	Actual (miles)	Goal (miles)	Actual (miles)	Goal (miles)	Actual (miles)	Goal (miles)	Actual (miles)
Off		2		4		14	
Off		3		4		16	
Off		3		5		18	
Off		3		6		20	
Off		3		7		20	
Off		3		8		20	
Off		2		4		16	
1		Off		Race Day*		10	
mile				10 Km.		(plus race)	

*Record race result page 152.

Beginner marathoner

The difference between the novice marathon runner and the marathoner who has completed several races at that distance is a matter of training, preparation, and experience. Training is the dues every marathon runner pays. Nowhere else is training so closely linked to racing. The difference between finishing and not finishing, between running the marathon in four hours or three, will be found right here in your *Training Diary* —in the record you keep of your daily, weekly, monthly mileage totals.

Marathon mania is sweeping the country. There are some 70,000 marathon runners in the United States alone. More than 5,000 of them qualified for Boston in 1978, and 5,000 to 10,000 prepared for marathons in Chicago, Honolulu, and New York. The classic distance of 26 miles, 385 yards, increasingly attracts runners of all ages. It is an exciting run—when you are properly prepared.

The Runner's Handbook details marathon training, Ken Young's "collapse point" theory, racing diets and carbohydrate loading, training guidelines and strategy. But here are some general tips for the beginner:

- The beginner marathoner should build his or her races toward the marathon. That is, run a few races of 10 kilometers to 10 miles, then a half-marathon to 20 miles about one to two months before your first marathon. Run at your approximate marathon pace goal, or slightly faster.
- Set a realistic marathon goal. Basically, that should be to train well, and finish.
- Keep a detailed training log.
- Eat properly. Novice marathoners should not experiment with the depletion cycle of the carbohydrate-loading process. You should consume more carbohydrates than proteins during the last three or four days before the race. But don't overeat or sharply change your diet. On race day, don't eat within two to four hours before the start.
- Drink fluids regularly during the race, even if it isn't a warm day and you aren't thirsty. Don't drink too much or take liquids other than water if you aren't used to them. Stop to drink or drink while slowly walking. You should not be in a hurry.
- Wear broken-in training shoes with good cushioning. Racing shoes are not necessary.
- Dress in layers if it is cold, or in loose, reflective clothing if hot (see Seasonal Tips on pages 32-35).

- Get up two or three hours, or more, before the race. Stretch for 15 minutes half an hour before the start. Do some walking and jogging to loosen up.
- Remember to Warm-up and Cool-down before all training sessions and the race.
- Line up in the middle or back of the pack so you won't get in the competitors' way and won't start too fast. Set a slow, comfortable pace. Restrain yourself. In the end, you may wish to alternate jogging with brisk walking. Keep moving.

Beginner marathoner's chart

How to use it. If you have been running 20 miles a week for two months or more, and there are still several months before the marathon you wish to enter, the following chart and guidelines will get you there. The chart and guidelines are flexible; use them as models, or follow them as closely as you wish. Enter your actual mileage next to the goals.

- Build your mileage gradually, not more than 10 percent of your weekly mileage per week.
- The chart suggests one long run, one medium run, three average runs, and one day off per week. Note that long runs (Sunday) are followed by days off (Monday). On that day off, stretch and walk. Take time to recover from your long training runs.
- Reach the 40-to-70-miles-per-week level at least two months before the marathon. Following the rule set forth for beginner racers, you should run twice the marathon distance, or 52 miles, as a basic, minimum level every week. A better weekly mileage would be 60 to 65 miles. Young's "collapse point" suggests totaling 63 miles per week.
- At least two months before the marathon, you should complete two long runs of 15 to 20 miles. The chart shows the point in your training that these runs should occur.
- Your pace should be LSD: long, slow distance at marathon race pace.
- The last two weeks of training should be light. Let your body rest for the big effort. Cut your mileage by 10 to 30 percent two weeks before the race, and by another 10 to 30 percent one week before the marathon. (For example, from 40 to 30 to 20 miles.) Take the last two days off, or jog short distances.

Recovery after the race includes hot baths, walks, stretching as soon as possible. Continue for several days. Gradually return to your regular running routine.

Competitive runner

The competitive runner may specialize in distances of 4 to 10 miles, or be a marathon addict, or run a variety of races. He or she is the most serious of runners. This competitor logs between 60 and 100 miles per week including one long run and one or two interval training sessions.

To reach this level, first build up a base of several months of 40 to 50 miles per week. Remember, increase your mileage only about 10 percent per week. Also, the Warm-up and Cool-down stretching is even more important now because you are putting your body under greater stress.

You need to build a sufficient weekly mileage base for the distance of the race; regular long runs to build endurance and anaerobic work to improve your ability to run fast; regular recovery days; regular races (two, but no more than three, a month), covering not more than 10 percent of your weekly training mileage; peak and recovery for races.

Beginner marathoner's four-month build-

Week	Monday		Tuesday		Wednesday		Thursday	
	Goal	Actual	Goal (miles)	Actual (miles)	Goal (miles)	Actual (miles)	Goal (miles)	Actual (miles)
1	Off		3		4		3	
2	Off		3		4		3	
3	Off		3		5		3	
4	Off		3		5		3	
5	Off		3		5		3	
6	Off		3		6		3	
7	Off		3		6		3	
8	Off		4		10		4	
9	Off		4		8		4	
10	Off		6		12		4	
11	Off		4		12		4	
12	Off		8		12		4	
13	Off		6		12		4	
14	Off		6		10		4	
15	Off		4		15		3	
16	Off		8		6		4	
(Race Week)								

Competitive runner's chart

How to use it. The chart is a guide. Adapt it to your training schedule, or follow it as closely as you wish. Note the alternate hard and easy days; easy means recovery, when you run with friends or fill in weekly mileage. Long days are runs of 15 to 30 miles, essential for marathon training.

Intense days involve a variety of workouts:

- *Races.* Race frequently, using races as part of your training. Or race sparingly and peak for all-out efforts. Don't over-race.
- *Fartlek* ("Speed play"). Runs in bursts; for example, a 12-mile workout would include a 3-mile jog, 6 miles of fartlek bursts, ending with a 3-mile jog. Bursts are of 50 yards to 1.5 miles. Recovery and work pace vary, but workout is intense.

up and taper program

Friday Goal (miles)	Friday Actual (miles)	Saturday Goal (miles)	Saturday Actual (miles)	Sunday Goal (miles)	Sunday Actual (miles)	TOTALS Goal (miles)	TOTALS Actual (miles)
3		3		6		22	
4		2		8		24	
5		2		8		26	
5		2		10		28	
5		3		12		31	
5		3		14		34	
6		3		16		37	
6		4		12		40	
5		3		20		44	
8		4		14		48	
6		4		20		52	
8		6		14		52	
6		4		20		52	
6		4		12		42	
4		4		10		40	
Off		2		Race Day		20	
				Marathon*		(plus race)	

*Record race result page 152.

- *Hard Pace*. Conditions you to hold a fast pace for an extended period. Example: a 3- to 4-mile jog, a run at near race pace for 4 to 6 miles, then a 2- or 3-mile jog.

- *Long intervals*. Trains the body for longer races. Builds confidence and strength. All workouts are preceded and followed by 2- to 4-mile jog. Example: four to eight 880-yard workouts at race pace; 440-yard recovery jog.

- *Short Intervals*. Builds anaerobic endurance for shorter races. Jog 2 to 4 miles before and after intense sessions. Example: alternate 440 yards and 220 yards, 440 followed by 110-yard recovery, 220 followed by 220-yard recovery. Repeat each set three to five times at race pace or faster.

- *Hill Training*. Strengthens the quadriceps, improves anaerobic endurance. Downhills teach proper form by improving stride and relaxation. Example: 50-yard hills. Charge hill at three-quarter effort for 30 to 50 yards into hill; continue running 15 to 20 yards over crest of hill. Jog back down. Do six to twelve repetitions.

Monday	Tuesday	Wednesday	Thursday	Friday	Saturday	Sunday
Easy day 5-10 miles	Long 15-30	Easy 5-10	Intense 10	Easy 5-10	Easy 5-10	Intense 10-15

Here are some training guidelines:

- To break up existing mileage, or to add mileage, try running twice a day, early morning and evening.

- Competitors should not run more than two intense workouts a week, combined with one long run. Advanced competitors may run up to three.

- Stretch and warm up 15 minutes before all runs. Jog 2 or 3 miles before intense workouts, and cool down with a 2- or 3-mile jog. Stretch for 10 minutes afterward.

- Recovery pulse for interval runs should be below 120 beats per minute before starting next interval; take more recovery time if needed.

- Paces and recovery times for speed workouts are flexible. They will vary from runner to runner, and even day to day.

- As you become more fit, increase your pace, cut back your recovery time, increase your repetitions.

- Ease into these workouts.

- Take an extra recovery day after intense workouts, if needed.

Goals

Everyone who runs should have goals. At first, running itself is enough of a goal. Or you may want to get thinner, run longer, enter more races, place better. Each runner should set modest, attainable, yet challenging goals. Here are some suggestions:

- Beginner runner: To run comfortably for 20 consecutive minutes at a time, three to five days a week.
- Intermediate runner: To keep fit, to run easily 30 minutes a day at least five days a week, and to increase your distance.
- Beginner racer: To finish your first race without strain.
- Beginner marathoner: To finish the race in good health.
- Competitor: To maintain your high level of fitness, and to improve your race results at a variety of distances.

Whatever your personal goals, put them in this *Training Diary* so that you can look back in twelve months and say, "I'm going to do better than last year."

Clothes/equipment

Shoes. The most important investment a runner makes—and the most expensive—is a pair of well-cushioned running shoes. Sneakers and cheap imitations are not acceptable and may cause foot injury. *The Runner's Handbook* has an entire chapter, with diagrams, on shoes.

Try on your running shoes in the shop. Find a pair that feels comfortable. If one style and make feel good, but the sole is uncomfortable (the cleat or disk sits under the ball of your foot, for instance), try another pair of the same style and make. Mass-produced shoes do vary. Be sure to try on the shoes while wearing the socks you run in; also, bring your arch supports or other inserts along and have them in place when you try on shoes.

Running shoes must be flexible—bend them—with a stable heel. Look for good padding under the entire foot, especially the heel where you land. Nylon uppers dry faster than leather, break in easier, and are washable.

Number your pairs of running shoes, and record the mileage and wear in this *Training Diary*. Also, check the shoes you plan to buy to be sure the balance (heel support) is vertical. A sloped balance may cause an uneven footstrike.

Worn running shoes can be resoled (see *The Runner's Handbook*, pages 212-214).

Socks. Socks can provide extra cushioning and they absorb sweat. In winter, wool socks will provide warmth even when wet. In summer, some runners prefer no socks, or anklets.

Clothing. Don't overdress or underdress. Your body builds heat rapidly as you run. Dress in loose-fitting clothing, in layers that can be unzipped or removed. Hats trap heat in winter and shade you in summer. Be sure to cover the ears and fingers in winter.

Diet

Many people run to lose weight or to hold their weight in check. Diet and exercise go together. Unused muscle tissue becomes fat; no one can lose weight and hold that loss without exercise.

Runners soon learn that if you exercise regularly and vigorously, you can ignore going on a diet. Your weight will stabilize. Food will be absorbed and used more efficiently. Remember: just because you start to run does not mean that you can also overeat.

Here are some diet guidelines:

- Watch your food intake, get regular exercise, avoid snacking.
- Avoid bacon, sausage, eggs, French-fried potatoes, cream and ice cream, bread and butter, desserts.
- Use jam instead of margarine, skim milk instead of whole milk.
- Stop using salt. Remove the salt shaker from your table. There are plenty of natural salts in and on food you eat.
- Stop consuming sugar. Avoid candy. Get sugars from fresh fruits.
- Eat small, light lunches.
- Cut way back on the amount of meat you consume, especially hamburgers and hot dogs.
- Eat more fish and poultry.
- Eat a good breakfast.
- Avoid coffee, nonherbal teas, and all soft drinks with sugar in them.

Drinks. Fluids are important to the runner. They replace salts and minerals lost during your workouts. About 20 minutes before you run, drink a glass or two of water, or try half orange juice, half water. Some runners drink slightly salted half-and-half orange juice and water. Others drink water with a slice of lemon in it. Remember: drink during your runs on hot days.

Vitamins. There are no special pills that make you a stronger, faster runner. The best advice is to eat carefully and well, drink plenty of fluids, and get 8 hours sleep a night. Some physicians recommend 500 to 1,000 milligrams of vitamin C daily. Others suggest other vitamins. If you are eating a balanced diet, you may not need vitamin supplements at all.

Tip. Try eating your meal 15 minutes or so after your workout. Your appetite is depressed, and you will eat less.

Men's Weight Chart

How to use it. Find your height in inches, multiply by 2. This is the average weight for world-class runners for that height. The ideal competitor's weight should be within 10 percent of this figure. Like all charts, consider this an estimate.

Height	Weight (pounds)		
	World class	Competitor	Average healthy man
5'4" (64")	128	141	155
5'5" (65")	130	143	157
5'6" (66")	132	145	160
5'7" (67")	134	147	162
5'8" (68")	136	149	164
5'9" (69")	138	152	167
5'10" (70")	140	154	169
5'11" (71")	142	156	172
6' (72")	144	158	174
6'1" (73")	146	160	176
6'2" (74")	148	163	179
6'3" (75")	150	165	181
6'4" (76")	152	167	183
6'5" (77")	154	169	185
6'6" (78")	156	171	187

Women's Weight Chart

How to use it. Women competitors should use the first weight in their range as an approximate goal. For example, a woman competitor 5 feet tall, with a small frame should weigh about 100 pounds. Women 18 to 25 should subtract 1 pound for each year under 25. *This chart is an estimate because women are new to competitive running.*

Height	Weight (pounds)		
	Small frame	Medium frame	Large frame
4'10"	92-98	96-107	104-119
4'11"	94-101	98-110	106-122
5'	96-104	101-113	109-125
5'1"	99-107	104-116	112-128
5'2"	102-110	107-119	115-131
5'3"	105-113	110-122	118-134
5'4"	108-116	113-125	121-138
5'5"	111-119	116-130	125-142
5'6"	114-123	120-135	129-146
5'7"	118-127	124-139	133-150
5'8"	122-131	128-143	137-154
5'9"	126-135	132-147	141-158
5'10"	130-140	136-151	145-163
5'11"	134-144	140-155	149-168
6'	138-148	144-159	153-173

Women and Running

Road running is the fastest growing sport in America, and it is growing fastest among women.

More than 1,000 women have now run the marathon distance (26 miles, 385 yards) in less than 4 hours.

Since 1969, the world marathon record for men has remained unbroken at 2:08:33. But during that same decade, women have dropped 33 minutes and 26 seconds off their world record, improving the time from 3:07:26 in 1969 to 2:34:37 in 1978.

Still, the longest Olympic distance that women are allowed (by men) to run is just 1,500 meters—less than a mile.

Ten reasons we get injured

1. **Weak feet.** Your foot strikes the ground 1,000 times during every 7- to 10-minute mile. The force of the impact is about three times your body weight. If your feet are weak, the force at footstrike strains the supporting tendons and muscles of the foot and leg. This often causes injury.

2. **Unequal leg length.** Fifteen percent of all runners have this problem. The result may be a series of hip, foot, leg, or back injuries. Heel lifts or inserts to balance the leg may help. Exercises to stretch and strengthen the affected areas are also beneficial.

3. **Poor flexibility.** Tight or shortened muscles are easily injured. Stretching, both before and after running, is essential to running injury-free.

4. **Weak antigravity muscles.** The back and leg muscles get overdeveloped with running. Strengthening exercises for the opposite group of muscles—abdominals, quadriceps, shins—are important.

5. **Stress and tension.** This is a cause of lower-back pain and injuries related to tense muscles forced into action. Relaxation exercises before and after running ease this problem.

6. **Overuse syndrome.** Overtraining, increasing your mileage by too much too soon, may cause injury. Overexertion symptoms include fatigue, chills, insomnia. Easing back on your schedule helps.

7. **Improper training habits.** Sudden changes in intensity, duration, or frequency of your runs should be avoided. So should sudden changes from dirt to hard pavement.

8. **Environmental factors.** Good running shoes are essential. Treat yourself to them. Also dress properly for the weather conditions.

9. **Injury rehabilitation.** Allow any injury to heal before returning to full workouts. Take time for recovery.

10. **Poor advice.** Be wary of nonathletic, out-of-shape doctors who prefer inactivity and pills as cures. Be even more wary of fellow runners who, after running a few miles a week, become "experts" in the field.

How to Return After Injury or Illness

Test yourself for a few days at half your average workout distance, or less. Take days off. Stretch a lot. Increase your mileage by only 10 to 20 percent until back to normal.

- Beware of relapse. Listen to your body.
- Be alert to favoring an injury. A slight limp, even blisters, can cause you to lean or favor the problem and cause injury elsewhere.

If you can't run after injury or illness:

- Work on stretching, weight training, and so forth, so you won't feel you are wasting time.
- Do cardiovascular work on a bicycle (if you can), swim, or walk. Work to maintain cardiovascular level, muscle strength, and flexibility.

Two weeks without running will set you back. A few days out is okay. Your body will rebel, but work it back slowly.

Seasonal tips: Cold weather

Some runners feel that fall and winter are the finest running seasons. Fall may be the best season of all, stretching from summer's heat to winter's chill. There will be days when you should review the lessons of summer running. And there will be enough cold days to warn you to prepare for runs in subfreezing weather.

Like spring, fall is a good time for planning. It is an excellent time for races. The pinnacle comes in September in Chicago and in October in the New York City Marathon. Or you may want to set fall and winter training schedules that lead to spring competitions—and Boston.

Here are some fall tips:

- In most parts of the northern hemisphere, fall means rain. Wet clothing extracts heat from your body up to 240 times as fast as dry clothing. The rains of autumn chill. Wool, however, even when wet, will keep you warm. Other fabrics create a "wicking" action that draws heat from your body and passes it into the air. Wear layers of clothing, including a warm cap or hat.
- Don't wear a rubber rainsuit. This traps dangerous levels of body heat and may cause dehydration.
- Yes, run in the rain. Get wet. You'll generate plenty of heat and your layers will keep you warm. Wear nylon shoes and nylon shorts, which dry fast. Avoid cotton shorts and sweatpants which get heavy and droop when wet. Rub Vaseline on your legs for protection, and wear shorts.
- After your run, change quickly into warm, dry clothing.
- Protect yourself from chilling fall winds with lightweight nylon or cotton windbreaker. Later, try a heavier sweatsuit with pouch pocket. A down vest will get you through late fall, and much of winter.

Don't let Father Winter keep you from running. Winter runs can be safe, enjoyable. Plan them carefully. Remember to warm-up and cool-down indoors.

Here are some tips for cold-weather running:

- *Snow:* Run in the stuff. Eat it. Let it fall upon you for insulation. Running in a light snowfall can be the best run of the four seasons. Footing is good, the ground has a special snow cushion to make your steps lighter, traction is solid. Listen to the soft "shush" of the falling flakes.
- *Wind:* Protect yourself against winter wind by selecting your running routes carefully, wearing proper clothing in layers.

If you run an out-and-back course, run first into the wind. This will avoid building up a sweat during the out leg and running into a chilling wind on the way back.

A ski mask will protect your face in very cold winds. Ski goggles will protect your eyes. Vaseline smeared over the face will also cut down on wind burns. Chapstick or other protectors should be applied to your lips.

A scarf over the mouth, or a ski mask without mouth opening, will protect your lips and warm inhaled air. Few runners, however, use either. They are restricting, and the danger of frostbite in your lungs is almost nil. The cold air is usually warmed by the body's passages.

- *Clothing*. Use the layer theory. Your body creates heat, and in winter your clothing traps this heat and warms you with it. Wear running clothes in layers to create pockets of heat. Allow for unzipping to let heat escape (to avoid overheating).

From the skin out, an example of good layering for running would be: running shorts (athletic supporter), T-shirt (bra), thermal underwear, wool socks, sweatsuit, scarf, windbreaker, hat, gloves, running shoes.

Mittens are best for the hands; they keep your fingers together and warm. Dr. George Sheehan wears old socks. Be sure that whatever you wear covers your wrists. Sweatsuits with pouch pockets allow you to remove your mittens or hat and store them for a while.

Protect your head. A hat or wool cap is essential in winter. As much as 50 percent of your body heat is lost through your head, as through a chimney.

If you get hot, remove your hat first, then your mittens. As you cool, replace them in opposite order.

Feet endure best. Wool running socks are excellent, and all you need. If you keep moving you won't get cold. Frank Shorter, for example, runs outdoors all winter. His feet have been frostbitten once: while skiing.

Seasonal tips: Warm weather

These are the seasons of races, good runs, and a wide variety of workouts. There are still chilly days left in spring, and there is the wilting heat of summer. During both seasons you may find yourself running in vacation areas such as beaches and mountains, as well as along your favorite paths.

Heat is the greatest problem of these seasons. Wherever you run, whatever your training level, here are some tips for warm-weather running:

- Try to avoid the hottest time of the day by running early in the morning or later in the evening.
- Look for shaded areas.
- Adjust your workouts. You may need to go slower and cut down on your distance, perhaps even dividing your running into morning and evening sessions.
- Drink plenty of fluids before, during, and after your runs. Water is best. Commercial drinks for runners are okay during races—if you are used to the beverages—although you'll find that many runners prepare and drink their own special brews. Runners lose salt and vitamin C through

sweating. A good substitute may be slightly salted orange juice thinned by adding half water. Avoid Cokes, iced tea or coffee, or diet drinks because of their sugar content. Sugar slows the body's absorption of water and creates a demand for more sugar.

Before you run, try drinking water or thinned orange juice. Or, 20 minutes before your workout, eat an orange. Drinking before running will not harm you, nor will drinking during your runs. Some runners, in fact, pace their hot-weather workouts from drinking fountain to drinking fountain. Dehydration—not drinking fluids—is a serious danger.

Remember: It takes 15 to 20 minutes for your body to absorb new fluids. Allow that time before you run, and then drink moderately as you go.

- Keep your body wet. Apply water to your head, neck, and upper body. Wet a handkerchief and cover your neck. Soak your running hat. Carry ice in your hands, or put it under your hat and let it melt.
- Wear light-colored, loose-fitting clothing that provides good ventilation.

Do not wear tank tops. You'll get sunburned. One runner's clever idea is to cut small circles in an old T-shirt, and wear that.

- Beware of the dangers of heat cramps, heat exhaustion, and the sometimes fatal onset of heat stroke. Chilling, throbbing pressure in the head, nausea, unsteadiness, dry skin, hair standing erect on chest and arms are all danger signals. Stop, get into the shade, drink fluids slowly.
- The best summer advice is: run slowly and wisely. Some days will be so bad that you will want to slow your pace sharply. Or you may be better off not running at all.

As the best winter runs come in the snow, perhaps the best summer runs come in the rain. A cooling sprinkle that falls during your mid-summer workout is a time of joy. The earth and air smell rich and fragrant, and the temperature is likely to be ten degrees or more cooler.

Beware of lightning. Do not even begin your workouts if there is lightning. If you are caught in a sudden lightning storm, take shelter in a building or car. If none is available, enter a grove of trees, and lie on the ground away from any single tree. Do not enter shallow caves or depressions along the sides of hills.

Remember: Run along the roadside facing on-coming traffic. But if you can, alternate sides of the road during your runs to avoid having the same foot land on the lower (shoulder) side of the roadway's slope. Beaches will be a problem for the same reason.

WEEK May 21 - 27, 1978

DAY Monday   Time _____   Weather _____

Pace/Type of Workout _____

Where Run _____   Shoes _____

Comments Day off - walked Companions _____
to work and back - ½ mile Distance or time _____
each way - legs tight.

DAY Tuesday   Time 8-8:30 a.m. Weather Cool, 50°

Pace/Type of Workout slow and easy alt. run - walk.

Where Run Central Park reservoir Shoes new shoes (new balance 320)

Comments 1 loop   legs OK, Companions neighbor - Sally Jones
feel bloated
TNG Pulse ave. = 141   Distance or time _____
recovery Pulse = 91   run 4 / walk 1 x 4 =
                        16 minutes of running

DAY Wednesday   Time _____   Weather _____

Pace/Type of Workout _____

Where Run _____   Shoes _____

Comments stomach cramps Companions _____
20 minutes of stretching Distance or time _____
                        off

DAY Thursday   Time noon - 12:30 p.m. Weather Humid, 70°

Pace/Type of Workout slow, alternate run - walk

Where Run Central Park reservoir Shoes N.B. 320 - feel good

Comments 1 loop started period in Companions alone.
A.M. feel weak and lousy Distance or time _____
had to walk 2nd half of   run 4 / walk 1 x 2 = 8 min.
schedule pulse up to 160   then walk 15 minutes

DAY _Friday_ Time _____ Weather _____

Pace/Type of Workout _____

Where Run _____ Shoes _____

Comments _feel better._ Companions _____

walk to work and back. Distance or time _____

_____ | _off_

DAY _Saturday_ Time _10 A.M._ Weather _warm , 65°_

Pace/Type of Workout _slow alt. run - walk_

Where Run _Central Park reservior_ Shoes _N.B. 320_

Comments _felt great !_ Companions _RRC class - 200 People_

very comfortable Distance or time _____

ready to increase | _run 4 - walk 1 × 4_

TNG pulse — 140 Ave | _16 minutes_
recovery — 88

DAY _Sunday_ Time _____ Weather _____

Pace/Type of Workout _____

Where Run _____ Shoes _____

Comments _stretching_ Companions _____

20 minutes. Distance or time _____

legs feel good | _off_

SUMMARY _felt much better_ | _40 minutes_

after period started. Total: Distance or time _____

menstrual cramps seem Weight _120 (lost 2 lbs. for week)_

less of a problem due to Resting Heart Rate _75_

exercise. Have been on program for 3 weeks now!

Tip. When training, take frequent rest pauses: walk or slow your pace, drink fluids, and stretch.

WEEK 6/5 - 6/11

DAY _Monday_ 6/5 Time _____ Weather _____

Pace/Type of Workout _____

Where Run _____ Shoes _____

Comments _Still tired after_ Companions _____
20 miler yesterday. Walked Distance or time _____
2 miles. Stretched 20 min.

OFF

DAY _Tuesday_ 6/6 Time _6-7 p.m._ Weather _Cool 50°_

Pace/Type of Workout _First 2 mi easy - last 4 mi brisk / 7:30 pace_

Where Run _Central Park - 1 loop of_ drive Shoes _Nike waffle (#1)_
Double sweats for heat tng.

Comments _Sluggish until_ Companions _Alone_
picked up pace. Right Distance or time _____
Shin tender

6 MILES

DAY _Wednesday_ 6/7 Time _6-7:30 p.m._ Weather _Rain 60°_

Pace/Type of Workout _Easy and steady / 8:00 pace_

Where Run _Riverside Course to bridge_ Shoes _Nike Waffle (#2)_

Comments _Shin better, concen-_ Companions _John Smith + Sam Jones_
trated on running erect, _Good conversation_
stretched more before - Distance or time _____
iced shin after.

10 MILES

DAY _Thursday_ 6/8 Time _6-7 a.m._ Weather _Warm 75°_

Pace/Type of Workout _Fartlek 440 + 880 bursts off 7 min. pace - 2 mile jog before and after 4 mile intense_

Where Run _Cental Park Reservoir_ Shoes _Nike Elite -- race shoe_

Comments _Felt very strong_ Companions _John Smith_
Psyched for race Sunday _(he really pushed me)_ Distance or time _____

8 MILES

DAY _Friday_ 6/9 Time _Noon_ Weather _Warm 80°_

Pace/Type of Workout _Slow (8 pace) 4 miles. Brisk (7 pace) last 2 miles._

Where Run _Riverside Park_ Shoes _Nike Waffle (#1)_

Comments _legs a little tight_ Companions _alone_

Shins OK Distance or time _____

6 MILES

DAY _Saturday_ 6/10 Time _10 a.m._ Weather _Warm 75°_

Pace/Type of Workout _Easy — 7:30_

Where Run _Central Park - 4 mi loop_ Shoes _Nike Waffle (#2)_

Comments _Feel ready!!_ Companions _Sat. a.m. RRC class_

Distance or time _____

4 MILES

DAY _Sunday_ 6/11 Time _10 a.m._ Weather _Warm 70°_

Pace/Type of Workout _5 mile split -- 35 min. Time 71:02 Place 501/1500_

Where Run _Newark, N.J. 10 mile RACE_ Shoes _Nike Elite - slight blister on_ _Jog one before, 3 after._

right foot

Comments _PR by 2 minutes! Strong_ Companions _—_

at start, weak in middle -- Distance or time _____

Finished Strong -- rolling hills

14 MILES

SUMMARY _4th week in row of_ _48 MILES_

40+ extra mileage and Fartlek Total: Distance or time _____

sessions paying off. Think Weight _154 (down 2 lbs)_

Sub 3:15 marathon possible Resting Heart Rate _58_

by October.

Note. April 17, 1978: Fritz Mueller of New York City set the American Masters (over 40 years old) record for the marathon at Boston. Time: 2:20:47.

Goals for the Year

One-Year Runner's Diary

WEEK

DAY _____ Time _____ Weather _____

Pace/Type of Workout _____

Where Run _____ Shoes_____

Comments _____ Companions _____

_____ Distance or time _____

_____

_____

DAY _____ Time _____ Weather _____

Pace/Type of Workout _____

Where Run _____ Shoes_____

Comments _____ Companions _____

_____ Distance or time _____

_____

_____

DAY _____ Time _____ Weather _____

Pace/Type of Workout _____

Where Run _____ Shoes_____

Comments _____ Companions _____

_____ Distance or time _____

_____

_____

DAY _____ Time _____ Weather _____

Pace/Type of Workout _____

Where Run _____ Shoes_____

Comments _____ Companions _____

_____ Distance or time _____

_____

_____

DAY _____ Time _____ Weather _____

Pace/Type of Workout _____

Where Run _____ Shoes _____

Comments _____ Companions _____

_____ Distance or time _____

_____

_____

DAY _____ Time _____ Weather _____

Pace/Type of Workout _____

Where Run _____ Shoes _____

Comments _____ Companions _____

_____ Distance or time _____

_____

_____

DAY _____ Time _____ Weather _____

Pace/Type of Workout _____

Where Run _____ Shoes _____

Comments _____ Companions _____

_____ Distance or time _____

_____

_____

SUMMARY _____

_____ Total: Distance or time _____

_____ Weight _____

_____ Resting Heart Rate _____

Tip. When training, take frequent rest pauses: walk or slow your pace, drink fluids, and stretch.

WEEK _____

DAY _____ Time _____ Weather _____

Pace/Type of Workout _____

Where Run _____ Shoes_____

Comments _____ Companions _____

_____ | Distance or time _____

_____ |

_____ |

DAY _____ Time _____ Weather _____

Pace/Type of Workout _____

Where Run _____ Shoes_____

Comments _____ Companions _____

_____ | Distance or time _____

_____ |

_____ |

DAY _____ Time _____ Weather _____

Pace/Type of Workout _____

Where Run _____ Shoes_____

Comments _____ Companions _____

_____ | Distance or time _____

_____ |

_____ |

DAY _____ Time _____ Weather _____

Pace/Type of Workout _____

Where Run _____ Shoes_____

Comments _____ Companions _____

_____ | Distance or time _____

_____ |

_____ |

DAY _____ Time _____ Weather _____

Pace/Type of Workout _____

Where Run _____ Shoes_____

Comments _____ Companions _____

_____ Distance or time _____

_____

_____

DAY _____ Time _____ Weather _____

Pace/Type of Workout _____

Where Run _____ Shoes_____

Comments _____ Companions _____

_____ Distance or time _____

_____

_____

DAY _____ Time _____ Weather _____

Pace/Type of Workout _____

Where Run _____ Shoes_____

Comments _____ Companions _____

_____ Distance or time _____

_____

_____

SUMMARY _____

_____ Total: Distance or time _____

_____ Weight _____

_____ Resting Heart Rate _____

Note. April 17, 1978: Fritz Mueller of New York City set the American Masters (over 40 years old) record for the marathon at Boston. Time: 2:20:47.

WEEK

DAY _____ Time _____ Weather _____

Pace/Type of Workout _____

Where Run _____ Shoes_____

Comments _____ Companions _____

_____ Distance or time _____

_____

DAY _____ Time _____ Weather _____

Pace/Type of Workout _____

Where Run _____ Shoes_____

Comments _____ Companions _____

_____ Distance or time _____

_____

DAY _____ Time _____ Weather _____

Pace/Type of Workout _____

Where Run _____ Shoes_____

Comments _____ Companions _____

_____ Distance or time _____

_____

DAY _____ Time _____ Weather _____

Pace/Type of Workout _____

Where Run _____ Shoes_____

Comments _____ Companions _____

_____ Distance or time _____

_____

DAY _____ Time _____ Weather _____

Pace/Type of Workout _____

Where Run _____ Shoes_____

Comments _____ Companions _____

_____ Distance or time _____

_____|

_____|

_____

DAY _____ Time _____ Weather _____

Pace/Type of Workout _____

Where Run _____ Shoes_____

Comments _____ Companions _____

_____ Distance or time _____

_____|

_____|

_____

DAY _____ Time _____ Weather _____

Pace/Type of Workout _____

Where Run _____ Shoes_____

Comments _____ Companions _____

_____ Distance or time _____

_____|

_____|

_____|_____

SUMMARY _____|

_____ Total: Distance or time _____

_____ Weight _____

_____ Resting Heart Rate _____

Tip. Follow Joe Henderson's advice: "Run longer before running faster."

WEEK _____

DAY _____ Time _____ Weather _____

Pace/Type of Workout _____

Where Run _____ Shoes_____

Comments _____ Companions _____

_____ Distance or time _____

_____

_____

DAY _____ Time _____ Weather _____

Pace/Type of Workout _____

Where Run _____ Shoes_____

Comments _____ Companions _____

_____ Distance or time _____

_____

_____

DAY _____ Time _____ Weather _____

Pace/Type of Workout _____

Where Run _____ Shoes_____

Comments _____ Companions _____

_____ Distance or time _____

_____

_____

DAY _____ Time _____ Weather _____

Pace/Type of Workout _____

Where Run _____ Shoes_____

Comments _____ Companions _____

_____ Distance or time _____

_____

_____

DAY _____ Time _____ Weather _____

Pace/Type of Workout _____

Where Run _____ Shoes_____

Comments _____ Companions _____

_____ Distance or time _____

_____

_____

DAY _____ Time _____ Weather _____

Pace/Type of Workout _____

Where Run _____ Shoes_____

Comments _____ Companions _____

_____ Distance or time _____

_____

_____

DAY _____ Time _____ Weather _____

Pace/Type of Workout _____

Where Run _____ Shoes_____

Comments _____ Companions _____

_____ Distance or time _____

_____

_____

SUMMARY _____

_____ Total: Distance or time _____

_____ Weight _____

_____ Resting Heart Rate _____

Note. November 24, 1894: The first 19-mile Thanksgiving Day race was held in Hamilton, Ontario, Canada. It is the oldest race in North America.

WEEK

DAY _____ Time _____ Weather _____

Pace/Type of Workout _____

Where Run _____ Shoes _____

Comments _____ Companions _____

_____ Distance or time _____

_____

_____

DAY _____ Time _____ Weather _____

Pace/Type of Workout _____

Where Run _____ Shoes _____

Comments _____ Companions _____

_____ Distance or time _____

_____

_____

DAY _____ Time _____ Weather _____

Pace/Type of Workout _____

Where Run _____ Shoes _____

Comments _____ Companions _____

_____ Distance or time _____

_____

_____

DAY _____ Time _____ Weather _____

Pace/Type of Workout _____

Where Run _____ Shoes _____

Comments _____ Companions _____

_____ Distance or time _____

_____

_____

DAY _____ Time _____ Weather _____

Pace/Type of Workout _____

Where Run _____ Shoes_____

Comments _____ Companions _____

_____ Distance or time _____

_____

_____

DAY _____ Time _____ Weather _____

Pace/Type of Workout _____

Where Run _____ Shoes_____

Comments _____ Companions _____

_____ Distance or time _____

_____

_____

DAY _____ Time _____ Weather _____

Pace/Type of Workout _____

Where Run _____ Shoes_____

Comments _____ Companions _____

_____ Distance or time _____

_____

_____

SUMMARY _____

_____ Total: Distance or time _____

_____ Weight _____

_____ Resting Heart Rate _____

Tip. To keep your house keys safe while you run, lace them up with your running shoes, or pin them to your shorts.

WEEK

DAY _____ Time _____ Weather _____

Pace/Type of Workout _____

Where Run _____ Shoes _____

Comments _____ Companions _____

_____ Distance or time _____

_____

DAY _____ Time _____ Weather _____

Pace/Type of Workout _____

Where Run _____ Shoes _____

Comments _____ Companions _____

_____ Distance or time _____

_____

DAY _____ Time _____ Weather _____

Pace/Type of Workout _____

Where Run _____ Shoes _____

Comments _____ Companions _____

_____ Distance or time _____

_____

DAY _____ Time _____ Weather _____

Pace/Type of Workout _____

Where Run _____ Shoes _____

Comments _____ Companions _____

_____ Distance or time _____

_____

DAY _____ Time _____ Weather _____

Pace/Type of Workout _____

Where Run _____ Shoes_____

Comments _____ Companions _____

_____ Distance or time _____

_____

_____

DAY _____ Time _____ Weather _____

Pace/Type of Workout _____

Where Run _____ Shoes_____

Comments _____ Companions _____

_____ Distance or time _____

_____

_____

DAY _____ Time _____ Weather _____

Pace/Type of Workout _____

Where Run _____ Shoes_____

Comments _____ Companions _____

_____ Distance or time _____

_____

_____

SUMMARY _____

_____ Total: Distance or time _____

_____ Weight _____

_____ Resting Heart Rate _____

Note. 490 B.C. Pheidippides ran 24 miles from the battlefield at Marathon to Athens to report the Greeks' victory over the Persians. He then fell dead.

WEEK

DAY _____ Time _____ Weather _____

Pace/Type of Workout _____

Where Run _____ Shoes _____

Comments _____ Companions _____

_____ Distance or time _____

_____

_____

DAY _____ Time _____ Weather _____

Pace/Type of Workout _____

Where Run _____ Shoes _____

Comments _____ Companions _____

_____ Distance or time _____

_____

_____

DAY _____ Time _____ Weather _____

Pace/Type of Workout _____

Where Run _____ Shoes _____

Comments _____ Companions _____

_____ Distance or time _____

_____

_____

DAY _____ Time _____ Weather _____

Pace/Type of Workout _____

Where Run _____ Shoes _____

Comments _____ Companions _____

_____ Distance or time _____

_____

_____

DAY _____ Time _____ Weather _____

Pace/Type of Workout _____

Where Run _____ Shoes_____

Comments _____ Companions _____

_____ Distance or time _____

_____

_____

DAY _____ Time _____ Weather _____

Pace/Type of Workout _____

Where Run _____ Shoes_____

Comments _____ Companions _____

_____ Distance or time _____

_____

_____

DAY _____ Time _____ Weather _____

Pace/Type of Workout _____

Where Run _____ Shoes_____

Comments _____ Companions _____

_____ Distance or time _____

_____

SUMMARY _____

_____ Total: Distance or time _____

_____ Weight _____

_____ Resting Heart Rate _____

Tip. All runners take 15 minutes to stretch, relax, and warm up, and 10 minutes
to stretch and cool down.

WEEK _____

DAY _____ Time _____ Weather _____

Pace/Type of Workout _____

Where Run _____ Shoes _____

Comments _____ Companions _____

_____ Distance or time _____

_____

_____

DAY _____ Time _____ Weather _____

Pace/Type of Workout _____

Where Run _____ Shoes _____

Comments _____ Companions _____

_____ Distance or time _____

_____

_____

DAY _____ Time _____ Weather _____

Pace/Type of Workout _____

Where Run _____ Shoes _____

Comments _____ Companions _____

_____ Distance or time _____

_____

_____

DAY _____ Time _____ Weather _____

Pace/Type of Workout _____

Where Run _____ Shoes _____

Comments _____ Companions _____

_____ Distance or time _____

_____

_____

DAY _____ Time _____ Weather _____

Pace/Type of Workout _____

Where Run _____ Shoes_____

Comments _____ Companions _____

_____ Distance or time _____

_____

_____

DAY _____ Time _____ Weather _____

Pace/Type of Workout _____

Where Run _____ Shoes_____

Comments _____ Companions _____

_____ Distance or time _____

_____

_____

DAY _____ Time _____ Weather _____

Pace/Type of Workout _____

Where Run _____ Shoes_____

Comments _____ Companions _____

_____ Distance or time _____

_____

SUMMARY _____

_____ Total: Distance or time _____

_____ Weight _____

_____ Resting Heart Rate _____

Note. The oldest runner at the 1978 Boston Marathon was Dr. Everett Ames. He was seventy-six and finished the 26-mile, 385-yard, race in 4:51:00.

WEEK

DAY _____ Time _____ Weather _____

Pace/Type of Workout _____

Where Run _____ Shoes _____

Comments _____ Companions _____

_____ Distance or time _____

_____

_____

DAY _____ Time _____ Weather _____

Pace/Type of Workout _____

Where Run _____ Shoes _____

Comments _____ Companions _____

_____ Distance or time _____

_____

_____

DAY _____ Time _____ Weather _____

Pace/Type of Workout _____

Where Run _____ Shoes _____

Comments _____ Companions _____

_____ Distance or time _____

_____

_____

DAY _____ Time _____ Weather _____

Pace/Type of Workout _____

Where Run _____ Shoes _____

Comments _____ Companions _____

_____ Distance or time _____

_____

_____

DAY _____ Time _____ Weather _____

Pace/Type of Workout _____

Where Run _____ Shoes_____

Comments _____ Companions _____

_____ Distance or time _____

_____|

_____|

DAY _____ Time _____ Weather _____

Pace/Type of Workout _____

Where Run _____ Shoes_____

Comments _____ Companions _____

_____ Distance or time _____

_____|

_____|

DAY _____ Time _____ Weather _____

Pace/Type of Workout _____

Where Run _____ Shoes_____

Comments _____ Companions _____

_____ Distance or time _____

_____|

_____|

SUMMARY _____

_____ Total: Distance or time _____

_____ Weight _____

_____ Resting Heart Rate _____

Tip. Sprinting at the end of your run is not recommended. Pace yourself evenly throughout your workout or race.

WEEK

DAY _____ Time _____ Weather _____

Pace/Type of Workout _____

Where Run _____ Shoes _____

Comments _____ Companions _____

_____ Distance or time _____

_____

_____

DAY _____ Time _____ Weather _____

Pace/Type of Workout _____

Where Run _____ Shoes _____

Comments _____ Companions _____

_____ Distance or time _____

_____

_____

DAY _____ Time _____ Weather _____

Pace/Type of Workout _____

Where Run _____ Shoes _____

Comments _____ Companions _____

_____ Distance or time _____

_____

_____

DAY _____ Time _____ Weather _____

Pace/Type of Workout _____

Where Run _____ Shoes _____

Comments _____ Companions _____

_____ Distance or time _____

_____

_____

DAY _____ Time _____ Weather _____

Pace/Type of Workout _____

Where Run _____ Shoes_____

Comments _____ Companions _____

_____ Distance or time _____

_____

_____

DAY _____ Time _____ Weather _____

Pace/Type of Workout _____

Where Run _____ Shoes_____

Comments _____ Companions _____

_____ Distance or time _____

_____

_____

DAY _____ Time _____ Weather _____

Pace/Type of Workout _____

Where Run _____ Shoes_____

Comments _____ Companions _____

_____ Distance or time _____

_____

_____

SUMMARY _____

_____ Total: Distance or time _____

_____ Weight _____

_____ Resting Heart Rate _____

Note. April 10, 1896: The first Olympic marathon was run at Athens from Marathon Bridge to Olympic Stadium (24.85 miles). Spiridon Louis won; he averaged 7:12 a mile.

WEEK

DAY _____ Time _____ Weather _____

Pace/Type of Workout _____

Where Run _____ Shoes _____

Comments _____ Companions _____

_____ Distance or time _____

_____

_____

DAY _____ Time _____ Weather _____

Pace/Type of Workout _____

Where Run _____ Shoes _____

Comments _____ Companions _____

_____ Distance or time _____

_____

_____

DAY _____ Time _____ Weather _____

Pace/Type of Workout _____

Where Run _____ Shoes _____

Comments _____ Companions _____

_____ Distance or time _____

_____

_____

DAY _____ Time _____ Weather _____

Pace/Type of Workout _____

Where Run _____ Shoes _____

Comments _____ Companions _____

_____ Distance or time _____

_____

_____

DAY _____ Time _____ Weather _____

Pace/Type of Workout _____

Where Run _____ Shoes_____

Comments _____ Companions _____

_____ Distance or time _____

_____

DAY _____ Time _____ Weather _____

Pace/Type of Workout _____

Where Run _____ Shoes_____

Comments _____ Companions _____

_____ Distance or time _____

_____

DAY _____ Time _____ Weather _____

Pace/Type of Workout _____

Where Run _____ Shoes_____

Comments _____ Companions _____

_____ Distance or time _____

_____

_____

SUMMARY _____

_____ Total: Distance or time _____

_____ Weight _____

_____ Resting Heart Rate _____

Tip. Don't pound on Mother Earth: run gently, run silently, run long.

DAY _____ Time _____ Weather _____

Pace/Type of Workout _____

Where Run _____ Shoes_____

Comments _____ Companions _____

_____ Distance or time _____

_____

_____

DAY _____ Time _____ Weather _____

Pace/Type of Workout _____

Where Run _____ Shoes_____

Comments _____ Companions _____

_____ Distance or time _____

_____

_____

DAY _____ Time _____ Weather _____

Pace/Type of Workout _____

Where Run _____ Shoes_____

Comments _____ Companions _____

_____ Distance or time _____

_____

_____

DAY _____ Time _____ Weather _____

Pace/Type of Workout _____

Where Run _____ Shoes_____

Comments _____ Companions _____

_____ Distance or time _____

_____

_____

DAY _____ Time _____ Weather _____

Pace/Type of Workout _____

Where Run _____ Shoes_____

Comments _____ Companions _____

_____ Distance or time _____

_____

_____

DAY _____ Time _____ Weather _____

Pace/Type of Workout _____

Where Run _____ Shoes_____

Comments _____ Companions _____

_____ Distance or time _____

_____

_____

DAY _____ Time _____ Weather _____

Pace/Type of Workout _____

Where Run _____ Shoes_____

Comments _____ Companions _____

_____ Distance or time _____

_____

_____

SUMMARY _____

_____ Total: Distance or time _____

_____ Weight _____

_____ Resting Heart Rate _____

Note. September 20, 1896: Thirty runners took the train to Stamford, Connecticut, and ran to Columbus Circle, a distance of 25 miles, for first New York City Marathon. Winning time: 3:25:55.6.

WEEK _____

DAY _____ Time _____ Weather _____

Pace/Type of Workout _____

Where Run _____ Shoes_____

Comments _____ Companions _____

_____ Distance or time _____

_____

_____

DAY _____ Time _____ Weather _____

Pace/Type of Workout _____

Where Run _____ Shoes_____

Comments _____ Companions _____

_____ Distance or time _____

_____

_____

DAY _____ Time _____ Weather _____

Pace/Type of Workout _____

Where Run _____ Shoes_____

Comments _____ Companions _____

_____ Distance or time _____

_____

_____

DAY _____ Time _____ Weather _____

Pace/Type of Workout _____

Where Run _____ Shoes_____

Comments _____ Companions _____

_____ Distance or time _____

_____

_____

DAY _____ Time _____ Weather _____

Pace/Type of Workout _____

Where Run _____ Shoes _____

Comments _____ Companions _____

_____ Distance or time _____

_____

_____

DAY _____ Time _____ Weather _____

Pace/Type of Workout _____

Where Run _____ Shoes _____

Comments _____ Companions _____

_____ Distance or time _____

_____

_____

DAY _____ Time _____ Weather _____

Pace/Type of Workout _____

Where Run _____ Shoes _____

Comments _____ Companions _____

_____ Distance or time _____

_____

_____

SUMMARY _____

_____ Total: Distance or time _____

_____ Weight _____

_____ Resting Heart Rate _____

Tip. Don't run in rubber sweatsuits, which trap heat and may cause dehydration.

WEEK _____

DAY _____ Time _____ Weather _____

Pace/Type of Workout _____

Where Run _____ Shoes _____

Comments _____ Companions _____

_____ Distance or time _____

_____

_____

DAY _____ Time _____ Weather _____

Pace/Type of Workout _____

Where Run _____ Shoes _____

Comments _____ Companions _____

_____ Distance or time _____

_____

_____

DAY _____ Time _____ Weather _____

Pace/Type of Workout _____

Where Run _____ Shoes _____

Comments _____ Companions _____

_____ Distance or time _____

_____

_____

DAY _____ Time _____ Weather _____

Pace/Type of Workout _____

Where Run _____ Shoes _____

Comments _____ Companions _____

_____ Distance or time _____

_____

_____

DAY _____ Time _____ Weather _____

Pace/Type of Workout _____

Where Run _____ Shoes_____

Comments _____ Companions _____

_____ Distance or time _____

_____

_____

DAY _____ Time _____ Weather _____

Pace/Type of Workout _____

Where Run _____ Shoes_____

Comments _____ Companions _____

_____ Distance or time _____

_____

_____

DAY _____ Time _____ Weather _____

Pace/Type of Workout _____

Where Run _____ Shoes_____

Comments _____ Companions _____

_____ Distance or time _____

_____

_____

SUMMARY _____

_____ Total: Distance or time _____

_____ Weight _____

_____ Resting Heart Rate _____

Note. September 4, 1977: Kim Merritt of Racine, Wisconsin, set the American record for women at the Nike–Oregon T.C. Marathon, Eugene, Oregon. Time: 2:37:19.

WEEK

DAY _____ Time _____ Weather _____

Pace/Type of Workout _____

Where Run _____ Shoes_____

Comments _____ Companions _____

_____ Distance or time _____

_____

DAY _____ Time _____ Weather _____

Pace/Type of Workout _____

Where Run _____ Shoes_____

Comments _____ Companions _____

_____ Distance or time _____

_____

DAY _____ Time _____ Weather _____

Pace/Type of Workout _____

Where Run _____ Shoes_____

Comments _____ Companions _____

_____ Distance or time _____

_____

DAY _____ Time _____ Weather _____

Pace/Type of Workout _____

Where Run _____ Shoes_____

Comments _____ Companions _____

_____ Distance or time _____

_____

DAY _____ Time _____ Weather _____

Pace/Type of Workout _____

Where Run _____ Shoes_____

Comments _____ Companions _____

_____ Distance or time _____

_____

_____

DAY _____ Time _____ Weather _____

Pace/Type of Workout _____

Where Run _____ Shoes_____

Comments _____ Companions _____

_____ Distance or time _____

_____

_____

DAY _____ Time _____ Weather _____

Pace/Type of Workout _____

Where Run _____ Shoes_____

Comments _____ Companions _____

_____ Distance or time _____

_____

_____

SUMMARY _____

_____ Total: Distance or time _____

_____ Weight _____

_____ Resting Heart Rate _____

Tip. Increase your training mileage only by 10 to 20 percent a week—and no more.

WEEK

DAY _____ Time _____ Weather _____

Pace/Type of Workout _____

Where Run _____ Shoes _____

Comments _____ Companions _____

_____ Distance or time _____

_____

_____

DAY _____ Time _____ Weather _____

Pace/Type of Workout _____

Where Run _____ Shoes _____

Comments _____ Companions _____

_____ Distance or time _____

_____

_____

DAY _____ Time _____ Weather _____

Pace/Type of Workout _____

Where Run _____ Shoes _____

Comments _____ Companions _____

_____ Distance or time _____

_____

_____

DAY _____ Time _____ Weather _____

Pace/Type of Workout _____

Where Run _____ Shoes _____

Comments _____ Companions _____

_____ Distance or time _____

_____

_____

DAY _____ Time _____ Weather _____

Pace/Type of Workout _____

Where Run _____ Shoes_____

Comments _____ Companions _____

_____ Distance or time _____

_____

_____

DAY _____ Time _____ Weather _____

Pace/Type of Workout _____

Where Run _____ Shoes_____

Comments _____ Companions _____

_____ Distance or time _____

_____

_____

DAY _____ Time _____ Weather _____

Pace/Type of Workout _____

Where Run _____ Shoes_____

Comments _____ Companions _____

_____ Distance or time _____

_____

_____

SUMMARY _____

_____ Total: Distance or time _____

_____ Weight _____

_____ Resting Heart Rate _____

Note. The best Fun Run may be Kanawaha (West Virginia) Valley's Five Mile Poker Run. At each mile you are handed a playing card. Best hand at the finish wins.

WEEK _____

DAY _____ Time _____ Weather _____

Pace/Type of Workout _____

Where Run _____ Shoes _____

Comments _____ Companions _____

_____ Distance or time _____

_____

_____

DAY _____ Time _____ Weather _____

Pace/Type of Workout _____

Where Run _____ Shoes _____

Comments _____ Companions _____

_____ Distance or time _____

_____

_____

DAY _____ Time _____ Weather _____

Pace/Type of Workout _____

Where Run _____ Shoes _____

Comments _____ Companions _____

_____ Distance or time _____

_____

_____

DAY _____ Time _____ Weather _____

Pace/Type of Workout _____

Where Run _____ Shoes _____

Comments _____ Companions _____

_____ Distance or time _____

_____

_____

DAY _____ Time _____ Weather _____

Pace/Type of Workout _____

Where Run _____ Shoes_____

Comments _____ Companions _____

_____ Distance or time _____

_____

_____

DAY _____ Time _____ Weather _____

Pace/Type of Workout _____

Where Run _____ Shoes_____

Comments _____ Companions _____

_____ Distance or time _____

_____

_____

DAY _____ Time _____ Weather _____

Pace/Type of Workout _____

Where Run _____ Shoes_____

Comments _____ Companions _____

_____ Distance or time _____

_____

_____

SUMMARY _____

_____ Total: Distance or time _____

_____ Weight _____

_____ Resting Heart Rate _____

Tip. If dogs bother you during your runs, mix a solution of half water, half ammonia in a toy pistol, and zap the yappers.

WEEK _____

DAY _____ **Time** _____ **Weather** _____

Pace/Type of Workout _____

Where Run _____ **Shoes** _____

Comments _____ **Companions** _____

_____ **Distance or time** _____

_____

_____

DAY _____ **Time** _____ **Weather** _____

Pace/Type of Workout _____

Where Run _____ **Shoes** _____

Comments _____ **Companions** _____

_____ **Distance or time** _____

_____

_____

DAY _____ **Time** _____ **Weather** _____

Pace/Type of Workout _____

Where Run _____ **Shoes** _____

Comments _____ **Companions** _____

_____ **Distance or time** _____

_____

_____

DAY _____ **Time** _____ **Weather** _____

Pace/Type of Workout _____

Where Run _____ **Shoes** _____

Comments _____ **Companions** _____

_____ **Distance or time** _____

_____

_____

DAY _____ Time _____ Weather _____

Pace/Type of Workout _____

Where Run _____ Shoes_____

Comments _____ Companions _____

_____ Distance or time _____

_____

_____

DAY _____ Time _____ Weather _____

Pace/Type of Workout _____

Where Run _____ Shoes_____

Comments _____ Companions _____

_____ Distance or time _____

_____

_____

DAY _____ Time _____ Weather _____

Pace/Type of Workout _____

Where Run _____ Shoes_____

Comments _____ Companions _____

_____ Distance or time _____

_____

_____

SUMMARY _____

_____ Total: Distance or time _____

_____ Weight _____

_____ Resting Heart Rate _____

Note. April 19, 1897: The BAA held the first Patriot's Day Marathon to honor
Paul Revere's ride in 1775, 24.7 miles from Metcalfe's Hill in Ashland to
Boston's Irvington Street Oval. Winning time: 2:55:10.

WEEK _____

DAY _____ Time _____ Weather _____

Pace/Type of Workout _____

Where Run _____ Shoes _____

Comments _____ Companions _____

_____ Distance or time _____

_____

_____

DAY _____ Time _____ Weather _____

Pace/Type of Workout _____

Where Run _____ Shoes _____

Comments _____ Companions _____

_____ Distance or time _____

_____

_____

DAY _____ Time _____ Weather _____

Pace/Type of Workout _____

Where Run _____ Shoes _____

Comments _____ Companions _____

_____ Distance or time _____

_____

_____

DAY _____ Time _____ Weather _____

Pace/Type of Workout _____

Where Run _____ Shoes _____

Comments _____ Companions _____

_____ Distance or time _____

_____

_____

DAY _____ Time _____ Weather _____

Pace/Type of Workout _____

Where Run _____ Shoes_____

Comments _____ Companions _____

_____ Distance or time _____

_____

_____

DAY _____ Time _____ Weather _____

Pace/Type of Workout _____

Where Run _____ Shoes_____

Comments _____ Companions _____

_____ Distance or time _____

_____

_____

DAY _____ Time _____ Weather _____

Pace/Type of Workout _____

Where Run _____ Shoes_____

Comments _____ Companions _____

_____ Distance or time _____

_____

_____

SUMMARY _____

_____ Total: Distance or time _____

_____ Weight _____

_____ Resting Heart Rate _____

Tip. Run erect, hands held loosely, arms between waistline and chest.

WEEK _____

DAY _____ Time _____ Weather _____

Pace/Type of Workout _____

Where Run _____ Shoes_____

Comments _____ Companions _____

_____ Distance or time _____

_____

_____

DAY _____ Time _____ Weather _____

Pace/Type of Workout _____

Where Run _____ Shoes_____

Comments _____ Companions _____

_____ Distance or time _____

_____

_____

DAY _____ Time _____ Weather _____

Pace/Type of Workout _____

Where Run _____ Shoes_____

Comments _____ Companions _____

_____ Distance or time _____

_____

_____

DAY _____ Time _____ Weather _____

Pace/Type of Workout _____

Where Run _____ Shoes_____

Comments _____ Companions _____

_____ Distance or time _____

_____

_____

DAY _____ Time _____ Weather _____

Pace/Type of Workout _____

Where Run _____ Shoes_____

Comments _____ Companions _____

_____ Distance or time _____

_____

_____

DAY _____ Time _____ Weather _____

Pace/Type of Workout _____

Where Run _____ Shoes_____

Comments _____ Companions _____

_____ Distance or time _____

_____

_____

DAY _____ Time _____ Weather _____

Pace/Type of Workout _____

Where Run _____ Shoes_____

Comments _____ Companions _____

_____ Distance or time _____

_____

_____

SUMMARY _____

_____ Total: Distance or time _____

_____ Weight _____

_____ Resting Heart Rate _____

Note. The marathon distance of 26 miles, 385 yards, was established at the 1908 Olympics in London to allow the Royal Family to see the start of the race from Windsor Castle and the finish at the Royal Box—precisely that distance.

WEEK _____

DAY _____ Time _____ Weather _____

Pace/Type of Workout _____

Where Run _____ Shoes _____

Comments _____ Companions _____

_____ Distance or time _____

_____

_____

DAY _____ Time _____ Weather _____

Pace/Type of Workout _____

Where Run _____ Shoes _____

Comments _____ Companions _____

_____ Distance or time _____

_____

_____

DAY _____ Time _____ Weather _____

Pace/Type of Workout _____

Where Run _____ Shoes _____

Comments _____ Companions _____

_____ Distance or time _____

_____

_____

DAY _____ Time _____ Weather _____

Pace/Type of Workout _____

Where Run _____ Shoes _____

Comments _____ Companions _____

_____ Distance or time _____

_____

_____

DAY _____ Time _____ Weather _____

Pace/Type of Workout _____

Where Run _____ Shoes_____

Comments _____ Companions _____

_____ Distance or time _____

_____

_____

DAY _____ Time _____ Weather _____

Pace/Type of Workout _____

Where Run _____ Shoes_____

Comments _____ Companions _____

_____ Distance or time _____

_____

_____

DAY _____ Time _____ Weather _____

Pace/Type of Workout _____

Where Run _____ Shoes_____

Comments _____ Companions _____

_____ Distance or time _____

_____

_____

SUMMARY _____

_____ Total: Distance or time _____

_____ Weight _____

_____ Resting Heart Rate _____

Tip. Remember to belly-breathe: As you run, inhale through your mouth and expand your belly at the same time.

WEEK _____

DAY _____ Time _____ Weather _____

Pace/Type of Workout _____

Where Run _____ Shoes _____

Comments _____ Companions _____

_____ Distance or time _____

_____

_____

DAY _____ Time _____ Weather _____

Pace/Type of Workout _____

Where Run _____ Shoes _____

Comments _____ Companions _____

_____ Distance or time _____

_____

_____

DAY _____ Time _____ Weather _____

Pace/Type of Workout _____

Where Run _____ Shoes _____

Comments _____ Companions _____

_____ Distance or time _____

_____

_____

DAY _____ Time _____ Weather _____

Pace/Type of Workout _____

Where Run _____ Shoes _____

Comments _____ Companions _____

_____ Distance or time _____

_____

_____

DAY _____ Time _____ Weather _____

Pace/Type of Workout _____

Where Run _____ Shoes_____

Comments _____ Companions _____

_____ Distance or time _____

_____

_____

DAY _____ Time _____ Weather _____

Pace/Type of Workout _____

Where Run _____ Shoes_____

Comments _____ Companions _____

_____ Distance or time _____

_____

_____

DAY _____ Time _____ Weather _____

Pace/Type of Workout _____

Where Run _____ Shoes_____

Comments _____ Companions _____

_____ Distance or time _____

_____

SUMMARY _____

_____ Total: Distance or time _____

_____ Weight _____

_____ Resting Heart Rate _____

Note. The first winning time for a 26 mile, 385 yard marathon was 2:55:18.4 at
the 1908 Olympics, set by John Hayes of the United States.

WEEK _____

DAY _____ Time _____ Weather _____

Pace/Type of Workout _____

Where Run _____ Shoes _____

Comments _____ Companions _____

_____ Distance or time _____

_____

DAY _____ Time _____ Weather _____

Pace/Type of Workout _____

Where Run _____ Shoes _____

Comments _____ Companions _____

_____ Distance or time _____

_____

DAY _____ Time _____ Weather _____

Pace/Type of Workout _____

Where Run _____ Shoes _____

Comments _____ Companions _____

_____ Distance or time _____

_____

DAY _____ Time _____ Weather _____

Pace/Type of Workout _____

Where Run _____ Shoes _____

Comments _____ Companions _____

_____ Distance or time _____

_____

DAY _____ Time _____ Weather _____

Pace/Type of Workout _____

Where Run _____ Shoes_____

Comments _____ Companions _____

_____ Distance or time _____

_____

DAY _____ Time _____ Weather _____

Pace/Type of Workout _____

Where Run _____ Shoes_____

Comments _____ Companions _____

_____ Distance or time _____

_____

DAY _____ Time _____ Weather _____

Pace/Type of Workout _____

Where Run _____ Shoes_____

Comments _____ Companions _____

_____ Distance or time _____

_____

_____

SUMMARY _____

_____ Total: Distance or time _____

_____ Weight _____

_____ Resting Heart Rate _____

Tip. Enjoy the passing scenery. Remember what Snoopy said: "Jogging . . . is good for your heart and your legs and your feet. It's also very good for the ground. It makes it feel needed."

WEEK _____

DAY _____ Time _____ Weather _____

Pace/Type of Workout _____

Where Run _____ Shoes_____

Comments _____ Companions _____

_____ Distance or time _____

_____

_____

DAY _____ Time _____ Weather _____

Pace/Type of Workout _____

Where Run _____ Shoes_____

Comments _____ Companions _____

_____ Distance or time _____

_____

_____

DAY _____ Time _____ Weather _____

Pace/Type of Workout _____

Where Run _____ Shoes_____

Comments _____ Companions _____

_____ Distance or time _____

_____

_____

DAY _____ Time _____ Weather _____

Pace/Type of Workout _____

Where Run _____ Shoes_____

Comments _____ Companions _____

_____ Distance or time _____

_____

_____

DAY _____ Time _____ Weather _____

Pace/Type of Workout _____

Where Run _____ Shoes _____

Comments _____ Companions _____

_____ Distance or time _____

_____

_____

DAY _____ Time _____ Weather _____

Pace/Type of Workout _____

Where Run _____ Shoes _____

Comments _____ Companions _____

_____ Distance or time _____

_____

_____

DAY _____ Time _____ Weather _____

Pace/Type of Workout _____

Where Run _____ Shoes _____

Comments _____ Companions _____

_____ Distance or time _____

_____

_____

SUMMARY _____

_____ Total: Distance or time _____

_____ Weight _____

_____ Resting Heart Rate _____

Note. April 17, 1978: John A. Kelley ran his forty-seventh Boston Marathon. He won the Boston in 1935 and 1945 and placed second seven times.

WEEK

DAY _____ Time _____ Weather _____

Pace/Type of Workout _____

Where Run _____ Shoes _____

Comments _____ Companions _____

_____ Distance or time _____

_____

_____

DAY _____ Time _____ Weather _____

Pace/Type of Workout _____

Where Run _____ Shoes _____

Comments _____ Companions _____

_____ Distance or time _____

_____

_____

DAY _____ Time _____ Weather _____

Pace/Type of Workout _____

Where Run _____ Shoes _____

Comments _____ Companions _____

_____ Distance or time _____

_____

_____

DAY _____ Time _____ Weather _____

Pace/Type of Workout _____

Where Run _____ Shoes _____

Comments _____ Companions _____

_____ Distance or time _____

_____

_____

DAY _____ Time _____ Weather _____

Pace/Type of Workout _____

Where Run _____ Shoes _____

Comments _____ Companions _____

_____ Distance or time _____

_____

_____

DAY _____ Time _____ Weather _____

Pace/Type of Workout _____

Where Run _____ Shoes _____

Comments _____ Companions _____

_____ Distance or time _____

_____

_____

DAY _____ Time _____ Weather _____

Pace/Type of Workout _____

Where Run _____ Shoes _____

Comments _____ Companions _____

_____ Distance or time _____

_____

_____

SUMMARY _____

_____ Total: Distance or time _____

_____ Weight _____

_____ Resting Heart Rate _____

Tip. Don't run on your toes. Gently land on your heels and roll forward to the balls of your feet.

WEEK _____

DAY _____ Time _____ Weather _____

Pace/Type of Workout _____

Where Run _____ Shoes _____

Comments _____ Companions _____

_____ Distance or time _____

_____

_____

DAY _____ Time _____ Weather _____

Pace/Type of Workout _____

Where Run _____ Shoes _____

Comments _____ Companions _____

_____ Distance or time _____

_____

_____

DAY _____ Time _____ Weather _____

Pace/Type of Workout _____

Where Run _____ Shoes _____

Comments _____ Companions _____

_____ Distance or time _____

_____

_____

DAY _____ Time _____ Weather _____

Pace/Type of Workout _____

Where Run _____ Shoes _____

Comments _____ Companions _____

_____ Distance or time _____

_____

_____

DAY _____ Time _____ Weather _____

Pace/Type of Workout _____

Where Run _____ Shoes_____

Comments _____ Companions _____

_____|Distance or time _____

_____|

_____|

DAY _____ Time _____ Weather _____

Pace/Type of Workout _____

Where Run _____ Shoes_____

Comments _____ Companions _____

_____|Distance or time _____

_____|

_____|

DAY _____ Time _____ Weather _____

Pace/Type of Workout _____

Where Run _____ Shoes_____

Comments _____ Companions _____

_____|Distance or time _____

_____|

_____|

SUMMARY _____|

_____ Total: Distance or time _____

_____ Weight _____

_____ Resting Heart Rate _____

Note. August 10, 1956: First Pike's Peak (14,111 feet) Marathon held; 7,700 feet vertical climb, 13 miles up and back. Now it's 28 miles round trip.

WEEK _____

DAY _____ Time _____ Weather _____

Pace/Type of Workout _____

Where Run _____ Shoes_____

Comments _____ Companions _____

_____ Distance or time _____

_____

_____

DAY _____ Time _____ Weather _____

Pace/Type of Workout _____

Where Run _____ Shoes_____

Comments _____ Companions _____

_____ Distance or time _____

_____

_____

DAY _____ Time _____ Weather _____

Pace/Type of Workout _____

Where Run _____ Shoes_____

Comments _____ Companions _____

_____ Distance or time _____

_____

_____

DAY _____ Time _____ Weather _____

Pace/Type of Workout _____

Where Run _____ Shoes_____

Comments _____ Companions _____

_____ Distance or time _____

_____

_____

DAY _____ Time _____ Weather _____

Pace/Type of Workout _____

Where Run _____ Shoes_____

Comments _____ Companions _____

_____ Distance or time _____

_____

_____

DAY _____ Time _____ Weather _____

Pace/Type of Workout _____

Where Run _____ Shoes_____

Comments _____ Companions _____

_____ Distance or time _____

_____

_____

DAY _____ Time _____ Weather _____

Pace/Type of Workout _____

Where Run _____ Shoes_____

Comments _____ Companions _____

_____ Distance or time _____

_____

_____

SUMMARY _____

_____ Total: Distance or time _____

_____ Weight _____

_____ Resting Heart Rate _____

Tip. Running should be at a conversational pace. Find a group of friends to run and talk with.

WEEK

DAY _____ Time _____ Weather _____

Pace/Type of Workout _____

Where Run _____ Shoes _____

Comments _____ Companions _____

_____ Distance or time _____

_____

_____

DAY _____ Time _____ Weather _____

Pace/Type of Workout _____

Where Run _____ Shoes _____

Comments _____ Companions _____

_____ Distance or time _____

_____

_____

DAY _____ Time _____ Weather _____

Pace/Type of Workout _____

Where Run _____ Shoes _____

Comments _____ Companions _____

_____ Distance or time _____

_____

_____

DAY _____ Time _____ Weather _____

Pace/Type of Workout _____

Where Run _____ Shoes _____

Comments _____ Companions _____

_____ Distance or time _____

_____

_____

DAY _____ Time _____ Weather _____

Pace/Type of Workout _____

Where Run _____ Shoes _____

Comments _____ Companions _____

_____ Distance or time _____

_____

_____

DAY _____ Time _____ Weather _____

Pace/Type of Workout _____

Where Run _____ Shoes _____

Comments _____ Companions _____

_____ Distance or time _____

_____

_____

DAY _____ Time _____ Weather _____

Pace/Type of Workout _____

Where Run _____ Shoes _____

Comments _____ Companions _____

_____ Distance or time _____

_____

_____

SUMMARY _____

_____ Total: Distance or time _____

_____ Weight _____

_____ Resting Heart Rate _____

Note. Abebe Bikila of Ethiopia is the only man to win the Olympic Marathon twice, in 1960 (Rome) and 1964 (Tokyo). Times: 2:15:16.2 and 2:12:11.2.

WEEK _____

DAY _____ Time _____ Weather _____

Pace/Type of Workout _____

Where Run _____ Shoes_____

Comments _____ Companions _____

_____ Distance or time _____

_____

_____

DAY _____ Time _____ Weather _____

Pace/Type of Workout _____

Where Run _____ Shoes_____

Comments _____ Companions _____

_____ Distance or time _____

_____

_____

DAY _____ Time _____ Weather _____

Pace/Type of Workout _____

Where Run _____ Shoes_____

Comments _____ Companions _____

_____ Distance or time _____

_____

_____

DAY _____ Time _____ Weather _____

Pace/Type of Workout _____

Where Run _____ Shoes_____

Comments _____ Companions _____

_____ Distance or time _____

_____

_____

DAY _____ Time _____ Weather _____

Pace/Type of Workout _____

Where Run _____ Shoes _____

Comments _____ Companions _____

_____ Distance or time _____

_____

_____

DAY _____ Time _____ Weather _____

Pace/Type of Workout _____

Where Run _____ Shoes _____

Comments _____ Companions _____

_____ Distance or time _____

_____

_____

DAY _____ Time _____ Weather _____

Pace/Type of Workout _____

Where Run _____ Shoes _____

Comments _____ Companions _____

_____ Distance or time _____

_____

_____

SUMMARY _____

_____ Total: Distance or time _____

_____ Weight _____

_____ Resting Heart Rate _____

Tip. Promote the theory: Runners make better lovers.

WEEK

DAY _____ Time _____ Weather _____

Pace/Type of Workout _____

Where Run _____ Shoes _____

Comments _____ Companions _____

_____ Distance or time _____

_____

_____

DAY _____ Time _____ Weather _____

Pace/Type of Workout _____

Where Run _____ Shoes _____

Comments _____ Companions _____

_____ Distance or time _____

_____

_____

DAY _____ Time _____ Weather _____

Pace/Type of Workout _____

Where Run _____ Shoes _____

Comments _____ Companions _____

_____ Distance or time _____

_____

_____

DAY _____ Time _____ Weather _____

Pace/Type of Workout _____

Where Run _____ Shoes _____

Comments _____ Companions _____

_____ Distance or time _____

_____

_____

DAY _____ Time _____ Weather _____

Pace/Type of Workout _____

Where Run _____ Shoes_____

Comments _____ Companions _____

_____ Distance or time _____

_____

_____

DAY _____ Time _____ Weather _____

Pace/Type of Workout _____

Where Run _____ Shoes_____

Comments _____ Companions _____

_____ Distance or time _____

_____

DAY _____ Time _____ Weather _____

Pace/Type of Workout _____

Where Run _____ Shoes_____

Comments _____ Companions _____

_____ Distance or time _____

_____

_____

SUMMARY _____

_____ Total: Distance or time _____

_____ Weight _____

_____ Resting Heart Rate _____

Note. April 19, 1966: Roberta Gibb Bengay became the first unofficial woman
finisher at the Boston Marathon. Her time—3:21:00—beat two-thirds of the
field of men.

WEEK _____

DAY _____ Time _____ Weather _____

Pace/Type of Workout _____

Where Run _____ Shoes_____

Comments _____ Companions _____

_____|Distance or time _____

_____|

_____|

DAY _____ Time _____ Weather _____

Pace/Type of Workout _____

Where Run _____ Shoes_____

Comments _____ Companions _____

_____|Distance or time _____

_____|

_____|

DAY _____ Time _____ Weather _____

Pace/Type of Workout _____

Where Run _____ Shoes_____

Comments _____ Companions _____

_____|Distance or time _____

_____|

_____|

DAY _____ Time _____ Weather _____

Pace/Type of Workout _____

Where Run _____ Shoes_____

Comments _____ Companions _____

_____|Distance or time _____

_____|

_____|

DAY _____ Time _____ Weather _____

Pace/Type of Workout _____

Where Run _____ Shoes _____

Comments _____ Companions _____

_____ Distance or time _____

_____

_____

DAY _____ Time _____ Weather _____

Pace/Type of Workout _____

Where Run _____ Shoes _____

Comments _____ Companions _____

_____ Distance or time _____

_____

_____

DAY _____ Time _____ Weather _____

Pace/Type of Workout _____

Where Run _____ Shoes _____

Comments _____ Companions _____

_____ Distance or time _____

_____

_____

SUMMARY _____

_____ Total: Distance or time _____

_____ Weight _____

_____ Resting Heart Rate _____

Tip. Be consistent in your running. Put miles in the bank. Record them here.

WEEK

DAY _____ Time _____ Weather _____

Pace/Type of Workout _____

Where Run _____ Shoes _____

Comments _____ Companions _____

_____ Distance or time _____

_____

DAY _____ Time _____ Weather _____

Pace/Type of Workout _____

Where Run _____ Shoes _____

Comments _____ Companions _____

_____ Distance or time _____

_____

DAY _____ Time _____ Weather _____

Pace/Type of Workout _____

Where Run _____ Shoes _____

Comments _____ Companions _____

_____ Distance or time _____

_____

DAY _____ Time _____ Weather _____

Pace/Type of Workout _____

Where Run _____ Shoes _____

Comments _____ Companions _____

_____ Distance or time _____

_____

DAY _____ Time _____ Weather _____

Pace/Type of Workout _____

Where Run _____ Shoes_____

Comments _____ Companions _____

_____ Distance or time _____

_____

DAY _____ Time _____ Weather _____

Pace/Type of Workout _____

Where Run _____ Shoes_____

Comments _____ Companions _____

_____ Distance or time _____

_____

DAY _____ Time _____ Weather _____

Pace/Type of Workout _____

Where Run _____ Shoes_____

Comments _____ Companions _____

_____ Distance or time _____

_____

_____

SUMMARY _____

_____ Total: Distance or time _____

_____ Weight _____

_____ Resting Heart Rate _____

Note. May 30, 1969: The men's world record for the marathon was set by Derek Clayton of Australia. Time: 2:08:33.6.

WEEK _____

DAY _____ Time _____ Weather _____

Pace/Type of Workout _____

Where Run _____ Shoes _____

Comments _____ Companions _____

_____ | Distance or time _____

_____ |

_____ |

DAY _____ Time _____ Weather _____

Pace/Type of Workout _____

Where Run _____ Shoes _____

Comments _____ Companions _____

_____ | Distance or time _____

_____ |

_____ |

DAY _____ Time _____ Weather _____

Pace/Type of Workout _____

Where Run _____ Shoes _____

Comments _____ Companions _____

_____ | Distance or time _____

_____ |

_____ |

DAY _____ Time _____ Weather _____

Pace/Type of Workout _____

Where Run _____ Shoes _____

Comments _____ Companions _____

_____ | Distance or time _____

_____ |

_____ |

DAY _____ Time _____ Weather _____

Pace/Type of Workout _____

Where Run _____ Shoes_____

Comments _____ Companions _____

_____ Distance or time _____

_____

_____

DAY _____ Time _____ Weather _____

Pace/Type of Workout _____

Where Run _____ Shoes_____

Comments _____ Companions _____

_____ Distance or time _____

_____

_____

DAY _____ Time _____ Weather _____

Pace/Type of Workout _____

Where Run _____ Shoes_____

Comments _____ Companions _____

_____ Distance or time _____

_____

SUMMARY _____

_____ Total: Distance or time _____

_____ Weight _____

_____ Resting Heart Rate _____

Tip. Don't run the same distance every day. Follow the hard-easy rule.

WEEK _____

DAY _____ Time _____ Weather _____

Pace/Type of Workout _____

Where Run _____ Shoes _____

Comments _____ Companions _____

_____ Distance or time _____

_____

_____

DAY _____ Time _____ Weather _____

Pace/Type of Workout _____

Where Run _____ Shoes _____

Comments _____ Companions _____

_____ Distance or time _____

_____

_____

DAY _____ Time _____ Weather _____

Pace/Type of Workout _____

Where Run _____ Shoes _____

Comments _____ Companions _____

_____ Distance or time _____

_____

_____

DAY _____ Time _____ Weather _____

Pace/Type of Workout _____

Where Run _____ Shoes _____

Comments _____ Companions _____

_____ Distance or time _____

_____

_____

DAY _____ Time _____ Weather _____

Pace/Type of Workout _____

Where Run _____ Shoes_____

Comments _____ Companions _____

_____ Distance or time _____

_____

_____

DAY _____ Time _____ Weather _____

Pace/Type of Workout _____

Where Run _____ Shoes_____

Comments _____ Companions _____

_____ Distance or time _____

_____

_____

DAY _____ Time _____ Weather _____

Pace/Type of Workout _____

Where Run _____ Shoes_____

Comments _____ Companions _____

_____ Distance or time _____

_____

SUMMARY _____

_____ Total: Distance or time _____

_____ Weight _____

_____ Resting Heart Rate _____

Note. July 31, 1976: Waldemar Cierpinski of East Germany set the Olympic Marathon record. Time: 2:09:55.

WEEK _____

DAY _____ Time _____ Weather _____

Pace/Type of Workout _____

Where Run _____ Shoes _____

Comments _____ Companions _____

_____ Distance or time _____

_____

_____

DAY _____ Time _____ Weather _____

Pace/Type of Workout _____

Where Run _____ Shoes _____

Comments _____ Companions _____

_____ Distance or time _____

_____

_____

DAY _____ Time _____ Weather _____

Pace/Type of Workout _____

Where Run _____ Shoes _____

Comments _____ Companions _____

_____ Distance or time _____

_____

_____

DAY _____ Time _____ Weather _____

Pace/Type of Workout _____

Where Run _____ Shoes _____

Comments _____ Companions _____

_____ Distance or time _____

_____

_____

DAY _____ Time _____ Weather _____

Pace/Type of Workout _____

Where Run _____ Shoes _____

Comments _____ Companions _____

_____ Distance or time _____

_____

DAY _____ Time _____ Weather _____

Pace/Type of Workout _____

Where Run _____ Shoes _____

Comments _____ Companions _____

_____ Distance or time _____

_____

DAY _____ Time _____ Weather _____

Pace/Type of Workout _____

Where Run _____ Shoes _____

Comments _____ Companions _____

_____ Distance or time _____

_____

_____

SUMMARY _____

_____ Total: Distance or time _____

_____ Weight _____

_____ Resting Heart Rate _____

Tip. Getting stale? Take a few days off from running to swim, ride a bike, map a new running route.

WEEK

DAY _____ Time _____ Weather _____

Pace/Type of Workout _____

Where Run _____ Shoes_____

Comments _____ Companions _____

_____ Distance or time _____

_____

_____

DAY _____ Time _____ Weather _____

Pace/Type of Workout _____

Where Run _____ Shoes_____

Comments _____ Companions _____

_____ Distance or time _____

_____

_____

DAY _____ Time _____ Weather _____

Pace/Type of Workout _____

Where Run _____ Shoes_____

Comments _____ Companions _____

_____ Distance or time _____

_____

_____

DAY _____ Time _____ Weather _____

Pace/Type of Workout _____

Where Run _____ Shoes_____

Comments _____ Companions _____

_____ Distance or time _____

_____

_____

DAY _____ Time _____ Weather _____

Pace/Type of Workout _____

Where Run _____ Shoes_____

Comments _____ Companions _____

_____ Distance or time _____

_____

_____

_____

DAY _____ Time _____ Weather _____

Pace/Type of Workout _____

Where Run _____ Shoes_____

Comments _____ Companions _____

_____ Distance or time _____

_____

_____

DAY _____ Time _____ Weather _____

Pace/Type of Workout _____

Where Run _____ Shoes_____

Comments _____ Companions _____

_____ Distance or time _____

_____

_____

SUMMARY _____

_____ Total: Distance or time _____

_____ Weight _____

_____ Resting Heart Rate _____

Note. Clarence Demrar won the Boston Marathon seven times: 1911, 1922, 1923, 1924, 1927, 1928, 1930.

WEEK _____

DAY _____ Time _____ Weather _____

Pace/Type of Workout _____

Where Run _____ Shoes _____

Comments _____ Companions _____

_____ Distance or time _____

_____

DAY _____ Time _____ Weather _____

Pace/Type of Workout _____

Where Run _____ Shoes _____

Comments _____ Companions _____

_____ Distance or time _____

_____

DAY _____ Time _____ Weather _____

Pace/Type of Workout _____

Where Run _____ Shoes _____

Comments _____ Companions _____

_____ Distance or time _____

_____

DAY _____ Time _____ Weather _____

Pace/Type of Workout _____

Where Run _____ Shoes _____

Comments _____ Companions _____

_____ Distance or time _____

_____

DAY _____ Time _____ Weather _____

Pace/Type of Workout _____

Where Run _____ Shoes _____

Comments _____ Companions _____

_____ Distance or time _____

_____

_____

DAY _____ Time _____ Weather _____

Pace/Type of Workout _____

Where Run _____ Shoes _____

Comments _____ Companions _____

_____ Distance or time _____

_____

_____

DAY _____ Time _____ Weather _____

Pace/Type of Workout _____

Where Run _____ Shoes _____

Comments _____ Companions _____

_____ Distance or time _____

_____

_____

SUMMARY _____

_____ Total: Distance or time _____

_____ Weight _____

_____ Resting Heart Rate _____

Tip. Use running as your time out. Don't bring the hurried pace of life into your running.

WEEK

DAY _____ Time _____ Weather _____

Pace/Type of Workout _____

Where Run _____ Shoes _____

Comments _____ Companions _____

_____ Distance or time _____

_____

_____

DAY _____ Time _____ Weather _____

Pace/Type of Workout _____

Where Run _____ Shoes _____

Comments _____ Companions _____

_____ Distance or time _____

_____

_____

DAY _____ Time _____ Weather _____

Pace/Type of Workout _____

Where Run _____ Shoes _____

Comments _____ Companions _____

_____ Distance or time _____

_____

_____

DAY _____ Time _____ Weather _____

Pace/Type of Workout _____

Where Run _____ Shoes _____

Comments _____ Companions _____

_____ Distance or time _____

_____

_____

DAY _____ Time _____ Weather _____

Pace/Type of Workout _____

Where Run _____ Shoes_____

Comments _____ Companions _____

_____ Distance or time _____

_____

_____

DAY _____ Time _____ Weather _____

Pace/Type of Workout _____

Where Run _____ Shoes_____

Comments _____ Companions _____

_____ Distance or time _____

_____

_____

DAY _____ Time _____ Weather _____

Pace/Type of Workout _____

Where Run _____ Shoes_____

Comments _____ Companions _____

_____ Distance or time _____

_____

_____

SUMMARY _____

_____ Total: Distance or time _____

_____ Weight _____

_____ Resting Heart Rate _____

Note. September 19, 1971: Beth Bonner and Nina Kuscsik, running the New York City Marathon in hilly Central Park, became the first women to break three hours. Times: 2:55:22 and 2:56:04 respectively.

WEEK _____

DAY _____ Time _____ Weather _____

Pace/Type of Workout _____

Where Run _____ Shoes _____

Comments _____ Companions _____

_____ Distance or time _____

_____

_____

DAY _____ Time _____ Weather _____

Pace/Type of Workout _____

Where Run _____ Shoes _____

Comments _____ Companions _____

_____ Distance or time _____

_____

_____

DAY _____ Time _____ Weather _____

Pace/Type of Workout _____

Where Run _____ Shoes _____

Comments _____ Companions _____

_____ Distance or time _____

_____

_____

DAY _____ Time _____ Weather _____

Pace/Type of Workout _____

Where Run _____ Shoes _____

Comments _____ Companions _____

_____ Distance or time _____

_____

_____

DAY _____ Time _____ Weather _____

Pace/Type of Workout _____

Where Run _____ Shoes _____

Comments _____ Companions _____

_____ Distance or time _____

_____

_____

DAY _____ Time _____ Weather _____

Pace/Type of Workout _____

Where Run _____ Shoes _____

Comments _____ Companions _____

_____ Distance or time _____

_____

_____

DAY _____ Time _____ Weather _____

Pace/Type of Workout _____

Where Run _____ Shoes _____

Comments _____ Companions _____

_____ Distance or time _____

_____

_____

SUMMARY _____

_____ Total: Distance or time _____

_____ Weight _____

_____ Resting Heart Rate _____

Tip. Rub Vaseline on your feet to prevent blisters, inside your bra or shirt to avoid irritation from rubbing, and inside your crotch to prevent chaffing.

WEEK

DAY _____ Time _____ Weather _____

Pace/Type of Workout _____

Where Run _____ Shoes _____

Comments _____ Companions _____

_____ Distance or time _____

_____

_____

DAY _____ Time _____ Weather _____

Pace/Type of Workout _____

Where Run _____ Shoes _____

Comments _____ Companions _____

_____ Distance or time _____

_____

_____

DAY _____ Time _____ Weather _____

Pace/Type of Workout _____

Where Run _____ Shoes _____

Comments _____ Companions _____

_____ Distance or time _____

_____

_____

DAY _____ Time _____ Weather _____

Pace/Type of Workout _____

Where Run _____ Shoes _____

Comments _____ Companions _____

_____ Distance or time _____

_____

_____

DAY _____ Time _____ Weather _____

Pace/Type of Workout _____

Where Run _____ Shoes _____

Comments _____ Companions _____

_____ Distance or time _____

_____

_____

DAY _____ Time _____ Weather _____

Pace/Type of Workout _____

Where Run _____ Shoes _____

Comments _____ Companions _____

_____ Distance or time _____

_____

_____

DAY _____ Time _____ Weather _____

Pace/Type of Workout _____

Where Run _____ Shoes _____

Comments _____ Companions _____

_____ Distance or time _____

_____

_____

SUMMARY _____

_____ Total: Distance or time _____

_____ Weight _____

_____ Resting Heart Rate _____

Note. No Olympic Marathon winners have also won the Boston Marathon. Challengers who failed include Abebe Bikila of Ethiopia and Frank Shorter of the United States.

WEEK

DAY _____ Time _____ Weather _____

Pace/Type of Workout _____

Where Run _____ Shoes_____

Comments _____ Companions _____

_____ Distance or time _____

_____

_____

DAY _____ Time _____ Weather _____

Pace/Type of Workout _____

Where Run _____ Shoes_____

Comments _____ Companions _____

_____ Distance or time _____

_____

_____

DAY _____ Time _____ Weather _____

Pace/Type of Workout _____

Where Run _____ Shoes_____

Comments _____ Companions _____

_____ Distance or time _____

_____

_____

DAY _____ Time _____ Weather _____

Pace/Type of Workout _____

Where Run _____ Shoes_____

Comments _____ Companions _____

_____ Distance or time _____

_____

_____

DAY _____ Time _____ Weather _____

Pace/Type of Workout _____

Where Run _____ Shoes _____

Comments _____ Companions _____

_____ Distance or time _____

_____

_____

DAY _____ Time _____ Weather _____

Pace/Type of Workout _____

Where Run _____ Shoes _____

Comments _____ Companions _____

_____ Distance or time _____

_____

_____

DAY _____ Time _____ Weather _____

Pace/Type of Workout _____

Where Run _____ Shoes _____

Comments _____ Companions _____

_____ Distance or time _____

_____

_____

SUMMARY _____

_____ Total: Distance or time _____

_____ Weight _____

_____ Resting Heart Rate _____

Tip. Dr. Joan Ullyot, M.D., states that women runners may want to wear a bra for comfort. But not wearing a bra will not cause sagging or breast problems from running.

WEEK _____

DAY _____ **Time** _____ **Weather** _____

Pace/Type of Workout _____

Where Run _____ **Shoes** _____

Comments _____ **Companions** _____

_____ **Distance or time** _____

_____

_____

DAY _____ **Time** _____ **Weather** _____

Pace/Type of Workout _____

Where Run _____ **Shoes** _____

Comments _____ **Companions** _____

_____ **Distance or time** _____

_____

_____

DAY _____ **Time** _____ **Weather** _____

Pace/Type of Workout _____

Where Run _____ **Shoes** _____

Comments _____ **Companions** _____

_____ **Distance or time** _____

_____

_____

DAY _____ **Time** _____ **Weather** _____

Pace/Type of Workout _____

Where Run _____ **Shoes** _____

Comments _____ **Companions** _____

_____ **Distance or time** _____

_____

_____

DAY _____ Time _____ Weather _____

Pace/Type of Workout _____

Where Run _____ Shoes _____

Comments _____ Companions _____

_____ Distance or time _____

_____|

_____|

DAY _____ Time _____ Weather _____

Pace/Type of Workout _____

Where Run _____ Shoes _____

Comments _____ Companions _____

_____ Distance or time _____

_____|

_____|

DAY _____ Time _____ Weather _____

Pace/Type of Workout _____

Where Run _____ Shoes _____

Comments _____ Companions _____

_____ Distance or time _____

_____|

_____|

SUMMARY _____

_____ Total: Distance or time _____

_____ Weight _____

_____ Resting Heart Rate _____

Note. March 19, 1978: The Avon First International Women's Marathon held in
the United States, in Atlanta, Georgia. Winner: Martha Cooksey of California.
Time: 2:46:16.

WEEK _____

DAY _____ Time _____ Weather _____

Pace/Type of Workout _____

Where Run _____ Shoes _____

Comments _____ Companions _____

_____ Distance or time _____

_____

DAY _____ Time _____ Weather _____

Pace/Type of Workout _____

Where Run _____ Shoes _____

Comments _____ Companions _____

_____ Distance or time _____

_____

DAY _____ Time _____ Weather _____

Pace/Type of Workout _____

Where Run _____ Shoes _____

Comments _____ Companions _____

_____ Distance or time _____

_____

DAY _____ Time _____ Weather _____

Pace/Type of Workout _____

Where Run _____ Shoes _____

Comments _____ Companions _____

_____ Distance or time _____

_____

DAY _____ Time _____ Weather _____

Pace/Type of Workout _____

Where Run _____ Shoes_____

Comments _____ Companions _____

_____ Distance or time _____

_____

_____

DAY _____ Time _____ Weather _____

Pace/Type of Workout _____

Where Run _____ Shoes_____

Comments _____ Companions _____

_____ Distance or time _____

_____

_____

DAY _____ Time _____ Weather _____

Pace/Type of Workout _____

Where Run _____ Shoes_____

Comments _____ Companions _____

_____ Distance or time _____

_____

_____

SUMMARY _____

_____ Total: Distance or time _____

_____ Weight _____

_____ Resting Heart Rate _____

Tip. Off to the race? Remember to pack a small but adequate wad of toilet paper so you won't be caught without.

WEEK

DAY _____ Time _____ Weather _____

Pace/Type of Workout _____

Where Run _____ Shoes _____

Comments _____ Companions _____

_____ Distance or time _____

_____

_____

DAY _____ Time _____ Weather _____

Pace/Type of Workout _____

Where Run _____ Shoes _____

Comments _____ Companions _____

_____ Distance or time _____

_____

_____

DAY _____ Time _____ Weather _____

Pace/Type of Workout _____

Where Run _____ Shoes _____

Comments _____ Companions _____

_____ Distance or time _____

_____

_____

DAY _____ Time _____ Weather _____

Pace/Type of Workout _____

Where Run _____ Shoes _____

Comments _____ Companions _____

_____ Distance or time _____

_____

_____

DAY _____ Time _____ Weather _____

Pace/Type of Workout _____

Where Run _____ Shoes_____

Comments _____ Companions _____

_____ Distance or time _____

_____

_____

DAY _____ Time _____ Weather _____

Pace/Type of Workout _____

Where Run _____ Shoes_____

Comments _____ Companions _____

_____ Distance or time _____

_____

_____

DAY _____ Time _____ Weather _____

Pace/Type of Workout _____

Where Run _____ Shoes_____

Comments _____ Companions _____

_____ Distance or time _____

_____

SUMMARY _____

_____ Total: Distance or time _____

_____ Weight _____

_____ Resting Heart Rate _____

Note. May 1, 1977: Chantal Longlace of France set the women's world record for
the marathon: 2:35:15. Later that year, Christa Vahlensieck of West Germany
lowered that record: 2:34:37.

WEEK _____

DAY _____ Time _____ Weather _____

Pace/Type of Workout _____

Where Run _____ Shoes_____

Comments _____ Companions _____

_____ Distance or time _____

_____

_____

DAY _____ Time _____ Weather _____

Pace/Type of Workout _____

Where Run _____ Shoes_____

Comments _____ Companions _____

_____ Distance or time _____

_____

_____

DAY _____ Time _____ Weather _____

Pace/Type of Workout _____

Where Run _____ Shoes_____

Comments _____ Companions _____

_____ Distance or time _____

_____

_____

DAY _____ Time _____ Weather _____

Pace/Type of Workout _____

Where Run _____ Shoes_____

Comments _____ Companions _____

_____ Distance or time _____

_____

_____

DAY _____ Time _____ Weather _____

Pace/Type of Workout _____

Where Run _____ Shoes _____

Comments _____ Companions _____

_____ Distance or time _____

_____

_____

DAY _____ Time _____ Weather _____

Pace/Type of Workout _____

Where Run _____ Shoes _____

Comments _____ Companions _____

_____ Distance or time _____

_____

_____

DAY _____ Time _____ Weather _____

Pace/Type of Workout _____

Where Run _____ Shoes _____

Comments _____ Companions _____

_____ Distance or time _____

_____

_____

SUMMARY _____

_____ Total: Distance or time _____

_____ Weight _____

_____ Resting Heart Rate _____

Tip. To soothe that injury remember the old saw: Heat before/ice after.

DAY _____ Time _____ Weather _____

Pace/Type of Workout _____

Where Run _____ Shoes_____

Comments _____ Companions _____

_____ Distance or time _____

_____

_____

DAY _____ Time _____ Weather _____

Pace/Type of Workout _____

Where Run _____ Shoes_____

Comments _____ Companions _____

_____ Distance or time _____

_____

_____

DAY _____ Time _____ Weather _____

Pace/Type of Workout _____

Where Run _____ Shoes_____

Comments _____ Companions _____

_____ Distance or time _____

_____

_____

DAY _____ Time _____ Weather _____

Pace/Type of Workout _____

Where Run _____ Shoes_____

Comments _____ Companions _____

_____ Distance or time _____

_____

_____

DAY _____ Time _____ Weather _____

Pace/Type of Workout _____

Where Run _____ Shoes_____

Comments _____ Companions _____

_____ Distance or time _____

_____

_____

DAY _____ Time _____ Weather _____

Pace/Type of Workout _____

Where Run _____ Shoes_____

Comments _____ Companions _____

_____ Distance or time _____

_____

_____

DAY _____ Time _____ Weather _____

Pace/Type of Workout _____

Where Run _____ Shoes_____

Comments _____ Companions _____

_____ Distance or time _____

_____

_____

SUMMARY _____

_____ Total: Distance or time _____

_____ Weight _____

_____ Resting Heart Rate _____

Note. April 21, 1975: Bill Rodgers set the Boston and American marathon record of 2:09:55 — exactly the same time, to the very second, later set by Waldemar Cierpinski of East Germany in the 1976 Olympic Marathon.

WEEK _____

DAY _____ Time _____ Weather _____

Pace/Type of Workout _____

Where Run _____ Shoes _____

Comments _____ Companions _____

_____ Distance or time _____

_____

_____

DAY _____ Time _____ Weather _____

Pace/Type of Workout _____

Where Run _____ Shoes _____

Comments _____ Companions _____

_____ Distance or time _____

_____

_____

DAY _____ Time _____ Weather _____

Pace/Type of Workout _____

Where Run _____ Shoes _____

Comments _____ Companions _____

_____ Distance or time _____

_____

_____

DAY _____ Time _____ Weather _____

Pace/Type of Workout _____

Where Run _____ Shoes _____

Comments _____ Companions _____

_____ Distance or time _____

_____

_____

DAY _____ Time _____ Weather _____

Pace/Type of Workout _____

Where Run _____ Shoes_____

Comments _____ Companions _____

_____ Distance or time _____

_____

DAY _____ Time _____ Weather _____

Pace/Type of Workout _____

Where Run _____ Shoes_____

Comments _____ Companions _____

_____ Distance or time _____

_____

DAY _____ Time _____ Weather _____

Pace/Type of Workout _____

Where Run _____ Shoes_____

Comments _____ Companions _____

_____ Distance or time _____

_____

SUMMARY _____

_____ Total: Distance or time _____

_____ Weight _____

_____ Resting Heart Rate _____

Tip. Runners require extra vitamins that come from natural foods. Eat plenty of vegetables and fruits; drink a quart of water a day.

WEEK _____

DAY _____ Time _____ Weather _____

Pace/Type of Workout _____

Where Run _____ Shoes _____

Comments _____ Companions _____

_____ Distance or time _____

_____

_____

DAY _____ Time _____ Weather _____

Pace/Type of Workout _____

Where Run _____ Shoes _____

Comments _____ Companions _____

_____ Distance or time _____

_____

_____

DAY _____ Time _____ Weather _____

Pace/Type of Workout _____

Where Run _____ Shoes _____

Comments _____ Companions _____

_____ Distance or time _____

_____

_____

DAY _____ Time _____ Weather _____

Pace/Type of Workout _____

Where Run _____ Shoes _____

Comments _____ Companions _____

_____ Distance or time _____

_____

_____

DAY _____ Time _____ Weather _____

Pace/Type of Workout _____

Where Run _____ Shoes _____

Comments _____ Companions _____

_____ Distance or time _____

_____

_____

DAY _____ Time _____ Weather _____

Pace/Type of Workout _____

Where Run _____ Shoes _____

Comments _____ Companions _____

_____ Distance or time _____

_____

_____

DAY _____ Time _____ Weather _____

Pace/Type of Workout _____

Where Run _____ Shoes _____

Comments _____ Companions _____

_____ Distance or time _____

_____

_____

SUMMARY _____

_____ Total: Distance or time _____

_____ Weight _____

_____ Resting Heart Rate _____

Note. April 17, 1972: Nina Kuscsik became the first official woman winner of the Boston Marathon—76 years after first male winner. Time: 3:10:21.

WEEK _____

DAY _____ Time _____ Weather _____

Pace/Type of Workout _____

Where Run _____ Shoes _____

Comments _____ Companions _____

_____ Distance or time _____

_____

_____

DAY _____ Time _____ Weather _____

Pace/Type of Workout _____

Where Run _____ Shoes _____

Comments _____ Companions _____

_____ Distance or time _____

_____

_____

DAY _____ Time _____ Weather _____

Pace/Type of Workout _____

Where Run _____ Shoes _____

Comments _____ Companions _____

_____ Distance or time _____

_____

_____

DAY _____ Time _____ Weather _____

Pace/Type of Workout _____

Where Run _____ Shoes _____

Comments _____ Companions _____

_____ Distance or time _____

_____

_____

DAY _____ Time _____ Weather _____

Pace/Type of Workout _____

Where Run _____ Shoes_____

Comments _____ Companions _____

_____ Distance or time _____

_____

_____

DAY _____ Time _____ Weather _____

Pace/Type of Workout _____

Where Run _____ Shoes_____

Comments _____ Companions _____

_____ Distance or time _____

_____

_____

DAY _____ Time _____ Weather _____

Pace/Type of Workout _____

Where Run _____ Shoes_____

Comments _____ Companions _____

_____ Distance or time _____

_____

_____

SUMMARY _____

_____ Total: Distance or time _____

_____ Weight _____

_____ Resting Heart Rate _____

Tip. Walk before you jog, jog before you run. Mix walking and jogging, and gradually shift the proportions in favor of jogging as the weeks go by.

WEEK

DAY _____ Time _____ Weather _____

Pace/Type of Workout _____

Where Run _____ Shoes_____

Comments _____ Companions _____

_____ Distance or time _____

_____

_____

DAY _____ Time _____ Weather _____

Pace/Type of Workout _____

Where Run _____ Shoes_____

Comments _____ Companions _____

_____ Distance or time _____

_____

_____

DAY _____ Time _____ Weather _____

Pace/Type of Workout _____

Where Run _____ Shoes_____

Comments _____ Companions _____

_____ Distance or time _____

_____

_____

DAY _____ Time _____ Weather _____

Pace/Type of Workout _____

Where Run _____ Shoes_____

Comments _____ Companions _____

_____ Distance or time _____

_____

_____

DAY _____ Time _____ Weather _____

Pace/Type of Workout _____

Where Run _____ Shoes_____

Comments _____ Companions _____

_____ Distance or time _____

_____

_____

DAY _____ Time _____ Weather _____

Pace/Type of Workout _____

Where Run _____ Shoes_____

Comments _____ Companions _____

_____ Distance or time _____

_____

_____

DAY _____ Time _____ Weather _____

Pace/Type of Workout _____

Where Run _____ Shoes_____

Comments _____ Companions _____

_____ Distance or time _____

_____

_____

SUMMARY _____

_____ Total: Distance or time _____

_____ Weight _____

_____ Resting Heart Rate _____

Note. September 10, 1972: Frank Shorter won the Olympic Marathon in
2:12:9.8, and of his U.S. teammates, Kenny Moore placed fourth and Jack
Bachelor ninth. American marathon running boom got started.

Weekly mileage log

Week/ Date	Mileage	Weight	Resting Heart Rate*	Comments
1				
2				
3				
4				
5				
6				
7				
8				
9				
10				
11				
12				
13				

* Taken in bed before rising (see *The Runner's Handbook*, page 41-44).

Week/Date	Mileage	Weight	Resting Heart Rate	Comments
14				
15				
16				
17				
18				
19				
20				
21				
22				
23				
24				
25				
26				

148

Week/Date	Mileage	Weight	Resting Heart Rate	Comments
27				
28				
29				
30				
31				
32				
33				
34				
35				
36				
37				
38				
39				

Week/Date	Mileage	Weight	Resting Heart Rate	Comments
40				
41				
42				
43				
44				
45				
46				
47				
48				
49				
50				
51				
52				

Monthly mileage

Month	Miles	Comments
January		
February		
March		
April		
May		
June		
July		
August		
September		
October		
November		
December		

Summary of previous years

Year	Miles	Comments
19____		
19____		
19____		
19____		

Favorite running courses

How to use it. Record specific information on your favorite runs for future races. Below log good runs in other cities when you travel. Be sure to share these with other runners.

Location	Distance	Comments

Races of the year

Date	Event	Distance, Time/ Pace	Place/ Starters	Comments

Personal Records (PRs)

How to use it. Record your best-ever times for various races. Write in pencil so you can update as you get better.

Distance	Time	Date	Location/Comment
5 Km (3.1 miles)			
10 Km (6.2 miles)			
15 Km (9.3 miles)			
20 Km (12.4 miles)			
25 Km (15.5 miles)			
30 Km (18.6 miles)			
1 mile			
2 miles			
3 miles			
5 miles			
6 miles			
10 miles			
12 miles			
15 miles			
20 miles			
30 miles			
50 miles			
Half-marathon			
Marathon			
Other			

Marathon pacing chart

How to use it. This chart contains two sets of figures. On the left are hours; on the right, minutes per mile. Use the chart to set your pace goal per mile for the marathon. Also use it after the race to determine your average pace per mile.

To qualify for Boston, for example, men under 40 must run a marathon in three hours or better; that is a 6:51 per mile pace (3:00= 6:51:91). Women, and men over 40, must finish a marathon in 3½ hours or better; thus their pace is 3:30= 8:00:57 per mile.

2:00 = 4:34.61	2:30 = 5:43.26	3:00 = 6:51.91	3:30 = 8:00.57	4:00 = 9:09.24
2:01 = 4:36.90	2:31 = 5:45.55	3:01 = 6:54.20	3:31 = 8:02.86	4:01 = 9:11.53
2:02 = 4:39.18	2:32 = 5:47.84	3:02 = 6:56.49	3:32 = 8:05.15	4:02 = 9:13.82
2:03 = 4:41.47	2:33 = 5:50.13	3:03 = 6:58.78	3:33 = 8:07.44	4:03 = 9:16.11
2:04 = 4:43.76	2:34 = 5:52.41	3:04 = 7:01.07	3:34 = 8:09.73	4:04 = 9:18.40
2:05 = 4:46.05	2:35 = 5:54.70	3:05 = 7:03.36	3:35 = 8:12.02	4:05 = 9:20.69
2:06 = 4:48.34	2:36 = 5:56.99	3:06 = 7:05.64	3:36 = 8:14.31	4:06 = 9:22.98
2:07 = 4:50.63	2:37 = 5:59.28	3:07 = 7:07.93	3:37 = 8:16.60	4:07 = 9:25.27
2:08 = 4:52.92	2:38 = 6:01.57	3:08 = 7:10.22	3:38 = 8:18.89	4:08 = 9:27.56
2:09 = 4:55.20	2:39 = 6:03.86	3:09 = 7:12.51	3:39 = 8:21.18	4:09 = 9:29.85
2:10 = 4:57.49	2:40 = 6:06.15	3:10 = 7:14.80	3:40 = 8:23.46	4:10 = 9:32.13
2:11 = 4:59.78	2:41 = 6:08.43	3:11 = 7:17.09	3:41 = 8:25.75	4:11 = 9:34.42
2:12 = 5:02.07	2:42 = 6:10.72	3:12 = 7:19.38	3:42 = 8:28.04	4:12 = 9:36.71
2:13 = 5:04.36	2:43 = 6:13.01	3:13 = 7:21.67	3:43 = 8:30.33	4:13 = 9:39.00
2:14 = 5:06.65	2:44 = 6:15.30	3:14 = 7:23.96	3:44 = 8:32.62	4:14 = 9:41.29
2:15 = 5:08.93	2:45 = 6:17.59	3:15 = 7:26.25	3:45 = 8:34.91	4:15 = 9:43.58
2:16 = 5:11.22	2:46 = 6:19.88	3:16 = 7:28.54	3:46 = 8:37.20	4:16 = 9:45.87
2:17 = 5:13.51	2:47 = 6:22.16	3:17 = 7:30.83	3:47 = 8:39.59	4:17 = 9:48.16
2:18 = 5:15.80	2:48 = 6:24.45	3:18 = 7:33.12	3:48 = 8:41.88	4:18 = 9:50.45
2:19 = 5:18.09	2:49 = 6:26.74	3:19 = 7:35.41	3:49 = 8:44.17	4:19 = 9:52.74
2:20 = 5:20.38	2:50 = 6:29.03	3:20 = 7:37.68	3:50 = 8:46.35	4:20 = 9:55.02
2:21 = 5:22.66	2:51 = 6:31.32	3:21 = 7:39.97	3:51 = 8:48.64	4:21 = 9:57.31
2:22 = 5:24.95	2:52 = 6:33.61	3:22 = 7:42.26	3:52 = 8:50.93	4:22 = 9:59.60
2:23 = 5:27.24	2:53 = 6:35.89	3:23 = 7:44.55	3:53 = 8:53.22	4:23 = 10:01.89
2:24 = 5:29.53	2:54 = 6:38.18	3:24 = 7:46.84	3:54 = 8:55.51	4:24 = 10:04.18
2:25 = 5:31.82	2:55 = 6:40.47	3:25 = 7:49.13	3:55 = 8:57.80	4:25 = 10:06.47
2:26 = 5:34.11	2:56 = 6:42.76	3:26 = 7:51.42	3:56 = 9:00.09	4:26 = 10:08.76
2:27 = 5:36.40	2:57 = 6:45.05	3:27 = 7:53.71	3:57 = 9:02.38	4:27 = 10:11.05
2:28 = 5:38.68	2:58 = 6:47.34	3:28 = 7:56.00	3:58 = 9:04.67	4:28 = 10:13.34
2:29 = 5:40.97	2:59 = 6:49.63	3:29 = 7:58.29	3:59 = 9:06.96	4:29 = 10:15.63

Pacing chart

How to use it. Find a marked track or running path that covers 440 yards. Run it and time your pace. Check the chart to see what that would be per mile. For example, a 2-minute 440 is equivalent to an 8-minute mile. You can also determine your pace per mile. For example, to achieve a 36-minute run for 6 miles, you see on the chart that you must run 1 mile in 6 minutes, 2 in 12, 3 in 18, and so on. This will help you set even-pace goals for your races. Also, after a race, use the chart to check your race pace. For example, if you ran a 4-mile race (or training run) in 33:20, your pace was 8:30 per mile. (Time in the chart is in minutes and seconds.)

440 yards	Mile	2 miles	3 miles	4 miles	5 miles	6 miles
1:00	4:00	8:00	12:00	16:00	20:00	24:00
1:05	4:20	8:40	13:00	17:20	21:40	26:00
1:10	4:40	9:20	14:00	18:40	23:20	28:00
1:15	5:00	10:00	15:00	20:00	25:00	30:00
1:20	5:20	10:40	16:00	21:20	26:40	32:00
1:25	5:40	11:20	17:00	22:40	28:20	34:00
1:30	6:00	12:00	18:00	24:00	30:00	36:00
1:35	6:20	12:40	19:00	25:20	31:40	38:00
1:40	6:40	13:20	20:00	26:40	33:20	40:00
1:45	7:00	14:00	21:00	28:00	35:00	42:00
1:50	7:20	14:40	22:00	29:20	36:40	44:00	45:37
1:55	7:40	15:20	23:00	30:40	38:20	46:00	47:41
2:00	8:00	16:00	24:00	32:00	40:00	48:00	49:46
2:05	8:20	16:40	25:00	33:20	41:40	50:00	51:50
2:10	8:40	17:20	26:00	34:40	43:20	52:00
2:15	9:00	18:00	27:00	36:00	45:00	54:00
2:20	9:20	18:40	28:00	37:20	47:40	56:00
2:25	9:40	19:20	29:00	38:40	48:20	58:00
2:30	10:00	20:00	30:00	40:00	50:00	60:00

Mile-to-marathon chart

How to use it. This chart and the previous one overlap. You can check your training and race pace from 440 yards to the marathon (26 miles, 385 yards). This chart contains the most common racing distances and is based upon average pace per mile. If you are running a 15-mile race, for example, and wish to maintain a 7-minute pace, you must finish in 1 hour, 45 minutes (1:45:00). Use this chart also to determine your average race pace. Twenty miles run in 2:36:40 would equal a 7:50

mile pace. Notice, too, race splits at various distances and paces. These will help you set your pace.

Mile	5 Miles	10 Miles	15 Miles	20 Miles	Marathon
4:50	24:10	48:20	1:12:30	1:36:40	2:07:44
5:00	25:00	50:00	1:15:00	1:40:00	2:11:06
5:10	25:50	51:40	1:17:30	1:43:20	2:15:28
5:20	26:40	53:20	1:20:00	1:46:50	2:19:50
5:30	27:30	55:00	1:22:30	1:50:00	2:24:12
5:40	28:20	56:40	1:25:00	1:53:20	2:28:34
5:50	29:10	58:20	1:27:30	1:56:40	2:32:56
6:00	30:00	1:00:00	1:30:00	2:00:00	2:37:19
6:10	30:50	1:01:40	1:32:30	2:03:20	2:41:41
6:20	31:40	1:03:20	1:35:00	2:06:40	2:46:03
6:30	32:30	1:05:00	1:37:30	2:10:00	2:50:25
6:40	33:20	1:06:40	1:40:00	2:13:20	2:54:47
6:50	34:10	1:08:20	1:42:30	2:16:40	2:59:09
7:00	35:00	1:10:00	1:45:00	2:20:00	3:03:33
7:10	35:00	1:11:40	1:47:30	2:23:20	3:07:55
7:20	36:40	1:13:20	1:50:00	2:26:40	3:12:17
7:30	37:30	1:15:00	1:52:30	2:30:00	3:16:39
7:40	38:20	1:16:40	1:55:00	2:33:20	3:21:01
7:50	39:10	1:18:20	1:57:30	2:36:40	3:25:23
8:00	40:00	1:20:00	2:00:00	2:40:00	3:29:45
8:10	40:50	1:21:40	2:02:30	2:43:20	3:34:07
8:20	41:40	1:23:20	2:05:00	2:46:40	3:38:29
8:30	42:30	1:25:00	2:07:30	2:50:00	3:42:51
8:40	43:20	1:26:40	2:10:00	2:53:20	3:47:13
8:50	44:10	1:28:20	2:12:30	2:56:40	3:51:35
9:00	45:00	1:30:00	2:15:00	3:00:00	3:56:00
9:10	45:50	1:31:40	2:17:30	3:03:20	4:00:22
9:20	46:40	1:33:20	2:20:00	3:06:40	4:04:44
9:30	47:30	1:35:00	2:22:30	3:10:00	4:09:06
9:40	48:20	1:36:40	2:25:00	3:13:20	4:13:28
9:50	49:10	1:38:20	2:27:30	3:16:40	4:17:50
10:00	50:00	1:40:00	2:30:00	3:20:00	4:22:13

Metric pace chart

How to use it. If you enter a race measured in kilometers, this chart will help you determine your pace per mile. For example, if you run a 5-kilometer race in 19:10, by referring to the chart you can see that your pace was slightly more than 6:10 per mile. (Don't forget to enter your times on your Personal Record (PR) chart, page 153.)

You can also determine your race pace in advance for a kilometer race. If you are running a 10-kilometer race, and your goal is to do it at a 7-minute-per-mile pace, and the course is marked in kilometers, the chart shows that you should hit each kilometer mark at slightly faster than 4:21 per kilometer. The halfway mark would be slightly faster than 21:45.

The chart contains paces for 1, 5, and 10 kilometers. If you are running 15, 20, 25, or 30 kilometers, a little elementary arithmetic will find your pace. First, divide the kilometers run by 5. Next, take that answer and divide your time by it. Look up this time in the 5-kilometer column, and read over to the left for your pace per mile. For example, you ran a 20-kilometer race in 1:56:00. Divide 20 kilometers by five, which equals 4. Divide 1:56:00 by 4, and get 29 minutes. Take the chart, find 29 minutes under the 5-kilometer column, check left, and see that you ran the 20-kilometer race at a 9:20 per mile pace.

(Times on this chart are in minutes:seconds.tenths of seconds; example — 2:29.16).

Pace per mile	1 km	5 km	10 km
4:00	2:29.16	12:25.80	24:51.6
4:30	2:47.80	13:59.00	27:58.0
5:00	3:06.45	15:32.25	31:04.5
5:10	3:12.66	16:03.30	32:06.6
5:20	3:18.88	16:34.40	33:08.8
5:30	3:25.09	17:05.45	34:10.9
5:40	3:31.31	17:36.55	35:13.1
5:50	3:37.52	18:07.60	36:15.2
6:00	3:43.74	18:38.70	37:17.4
6:10	3:49.95	19:09.75	38:19.5
6:20	3:56.17	19:40.85	39:21.7
6:30	4:02.38	20:11.90	40:23.8
6:40	4:08.60	20.43.00	41:26.0
6:50	4:14.81	21:14.05	42:28.1
7:00	4:21.03	21:45.15	43:30.3
7:10	4:27.24	22:16.20	44:32.4
7:20	4:33.46	22:47.30	45:34.6
7:30	4:39.67	23:18.35	46:36.7
7:40	4:45.89	23:49.45	47:19.9
7:50	4:52.10	24:20.5	48:41.0
8:00	4:58.32	24:51.6	49:43.2
8:10	5:04.53	25:22.65	50:45.3
8:20	5:10.75	25:53.75	51:47.5
8:30	5:16.96	26:24.8	52:49.6
8:40	5:23.18	26:55.9	53:51.8
8:50	5:29.39	27:26.9	54:53.8
9:00	5:35.61	27:58.05	55:56.1
9:10	5:41.82	28:29.1	56:58.2
9:20	5:48.04	29:00.2	58:00.4
9:30	5:54.25	29:31.25	59:02.5
9:40	6:00.47	30:02.35	60:04.7
9:50	6:06.68	30:33.4	61:06.8
10:00	6:12.9	31:04.5	62:09.0

158

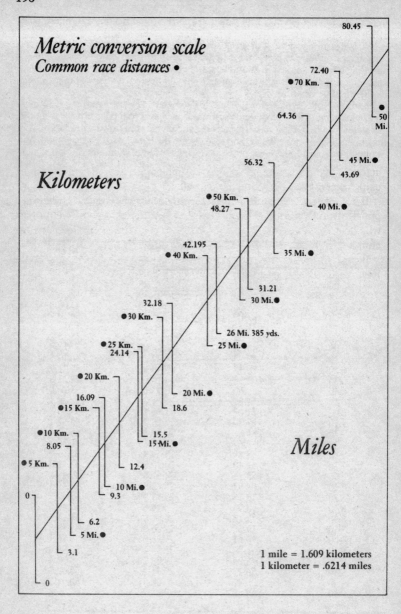

Metric conversion scale
Common race distances ●

Kilometers

Miles

80.45

72.40
● 70 Km.

64.36

50
Mi.

56.32

45 Mi. ●
43.69

● 50 Km.
48.27

40 Mi. ●

42.195
● 40 Km.

35 Mi. ●

31.21
30 Mi. ●

32.18
● 30 Km.

26 Mi. 385 yds.
25 Mi. ●

● 25 Km.
24.14

● 20 Km.

20 Mi. ●

16.09
● 15 Km.

18.6

● 10 Km.
8.05

15.5
15 Mi. ●

● 5 Km.

12.4

0

10 Mi. ●
9.3

6.2
5 Mi. ●

3.1

0

1 mile = 1.609 kilometers
1 kilometer = .6214 miles

Where to run when you're on the run

At one time or another, almost every runner will find himself or herself alone in a new city. Happily, running is a gregarious as well as healthy activity. There are runners and new running paths in almost every American city, and most foreign cities as well.

If you are a runner, and you travel, you have spent your last lonely days out of town. Better yet, you now have no excuse not to continue running when away on business or pleasure. This section details running paths and contacts in twenty-two American and six foreign cities.

Be sure to enter new running courses in your daily diary, and in the Favorite Courses log on page 151 of this *Training Diary*.

26 mi. 385 yds = 26.21875
13.10938

Where to run (in the United States)

Whatever your goals, here are some favorite running spots, and cities:

Atlanta

This is the "Running Capital of the South." Atlanta runners congregate at Phidippedes, owned by former Olympian Jeff Galloway.

Best runs: The downtown hotels are within two miles of Piedmont Park, with its woods, streets and golf course, and mounted police are around to protect joggers from nonjoggers.

Emory University, not far from Piedmont, is surrounded by neighborhoods filled with runners. Morningside and the Emory areas are favorites. Try the university's quarter-mile track, open to runners year round.

In Southwest Atlanta, Adams Park offers hilly running over a trail used by high-school cross-country teams. In the northwest, just off I-75, the Atlanta waterworks features two 1.2-mile courses that follow small lakes.

For a steep, 5-mile run, try Stone Mountain, fifteen miles west of Atlanta. The running path begins near the main parking lot.

Atlanta also offers a very popular "Peachtree" 10-kilometer run, held during the steamy July 4th weekend.

Running contacts:

YMCA (Downtown Branch), 145 Luckie St., NW, Atlanta, Ga. 30303; (404-525-5401).

The Atlanta Track Club, C/O Billy Daniel, 1760 Dyson Drive, NE, Atlanta, Ga. 30305.

Baltimore

Downtown visitors have several options. The Central YMCA on Franklin Street has a splendid elevated and banked indoor track. Or, you might want to take the historic run: Charles Street to Fort Avenue to Fort McHenry, a 6-mile run to the birthplace of the Star-Spangled Banner, with excellent views of the harbor.

Best runs: For hills, try Loch Raven Reservoir, over the city line on Loch Raven Blvd. From the parking lot near the dam to Dulaney Valley Road is about 3.5 miles. The toughest run in town is Satyr Hill, not far from Johns Hopkins University.

Herring Run Park offers a 1.35-mile flat course around Lake

Montebello. The city's bicyclists and joggers work out on a two-loop, two-mile cross-country path through hills and woods. The park's athletic fields also offer a flat, measured mile loop, broken into 100 yard distances for those wishing to do interval work.

Running contacts:

Every Sunday afternoon at two the Towson Branch of the YMCA sponsors a 1- and 2-mile Run for Your Life. (John Paletar, 301-256-1088).

The Baltimore Road Runners are also active on weekends throughout the year. They run 2 to 22 miles every Saturday morning at eight o'clock from the Loch Raven Dam. The start is actually in the lower Dam parking lot, one-third of a mile off Cromwell Bridge Road (301-668-3766).

The YMCA Central Branch, 24 Franklin St., Baltimore, Md. 21201; (301-539-7350). The Towson Family YMCA Branch, 600 W. Chesapeake Ave., Baltimore, Md. 21204; (301-823-8870).

Boston

Home of the Bean, the Cod, and the Marathon.

Boston is a runner's town, and features the world's most famous runner-bartender, Tommy Leonard. You can find him at Eliot's Lounge (Bill Rodgers' hangout), just around the corner·from the finish line in Boston. In 1977, Tommy held a carbohydrate-loading party for runners the day before the Marathon, and a glorious day-night after-the-race party. I think I remember something about that. Bill can also be found at his sports store on the course of the marathon at Cleveland Circle.

Best runs: The most pleasant runs may be along the Charles River. One, from the Prudential Center to Harvard University campus and back is about 10 miles. On the Cambridge side of the Charles is a wide path that is paved, flat and scenic. It is often filled with joggers. You can pick your distances by running along the Charles and looping across one of the many bridges.

Some distances: from Science Park to Watertown Square, 17 miles; to Eliot Bridge, 10 miles. At this bridge, turn to Fresh Pond, which *Runner's World* describes as "perhaps the most ideal running site around Boston." Run along Route 3 from the river. The paved path becomes 2.5 miles long by including the hill overlooking the parking lot. Distance markers are painted on the pavement.

Running from downtown hotels may be a problem. There is Boston Commons or the waterfront (Atlantic Avenue–Commercial Street), both pleasant during the day. Also, the park along the Charles on the Boston side by the Storrow Memorial Highway.

Long-distance runners who don't qualify for the Boston Marathon might want to pay homage to the infamous Newton Hills. Commonwealth Avenue in Newton covers three of the notorious four. Follow Lake Street to Newton Lower Falls; the return run totals 11 miles.

If you're on Cape Cod in August, try the scenic 7-mile run in Falmouth. In 1977, more than 2,000 runners made the trip.

Running contacts:

The Huntington Avenue Branch of the YMCA has an indoor track at 316 Huntington Ave., Boston, Mass., 02115; (617-536-7800).

The Road Runners put out *Yankee Runner* that covers New England. Write: Rick Bayko, 19 Grove Street, Merrimac, Mass. 01860; (617-346-9664).

The Greater Boston Track Club, Bill Rodgers' outfit, knows every path in the area. Try Bill Squires, 16 Crosby Road, Wakefield, Mass. 01880.

Women runners might want to check out the Liberty Athletic Club, which trains one of the top women's running teams in the U.S. Write—of all things—a man: John Babington, 4 Washington Avenue, Apt. 12A, Cambridge, Mass. 02140.

Chicago

The Windy City offers some fine runs along Lake Michigan.

Best runs: Lake Shore Drive, which follows the contour of the lake, is unmatched during warm weather. Between Foster Avenue Beach and the Museum of Science and Industry stretches 20.9 miles of sidewalk and path. Pick your distance and go running.

From most hotels around the Loop, a warm-up jog or brisk stroll brings you to Lake Shore Drive. From the University of Chicago, the Midway takes you directly to the beach.

There are also good parks and tracks. Riis Park, on Fullerton in the northwest section, holds races both winter and summer. There is a 400-meter cinder track. The fieldhouse, at last report, has working showers. Calumet Park, near the Indiana border, has a 4-mile loop and a lake view, while Washington and Jackson Parks near the University of Chicago have shorter loops. Both of these parks, however, should be avoided after dark. Stagg Field, near the university, offers a 440-yard Tartan track plus a larger oval track open for workouts between April and November.

Running contacts:

Lawson Center YMCA has a track at 30 W. Chicago Avenue, Chicago, Ill. 60616; (312-944-6211). The Tower YMCA (6300 W. Touhy, Niles, Ill. 60648; [312-744-8515]) also has an active fitness program.

The Mid-West Road Runners contact is Dick King, 500 So. Drexel, Chicago, Ill. 60606.

Cleveland

This is a tough city to run in, but also one filled with eager runners proud of the few fine courses available. Cleveland has cut itself off from its Lake Erie waterfront, but the persistent runner will find good runs there, and inland.

The city is ringed by an "emerald necklace" of parks in the suburbs that offer a variety of runs. Also, the long-distance runner can run from one park to another, with distances up to 20 miles.

In town, there is a track at Cleveland State University (at 30th Street between Euclid and Chester Avenues), near downtown hotels. Or take the Rapid Transit out as far as you wish (up to 5 miles), and run back along the trolley line on either pavement or the grass strip.

Best Run: From most hotels, head toward Public Square, the center of downtown Cleveland. Turn toward the lake on Ontario St. and head toward the waterfront parks. On Lakeside Avenue, turn right and run along Fort Huntington Park and Willard Park to East 9th Street. Turn left, toward the lake, for one block, cross the Amtrak lines, and look for the municipal parking lot on your right. Here is the start of a very good 7-mile run, most of it on grass, and the path of the Cleveland Marathon (which ends at Case Western Reserve in the suburbs).

The path starts in the parking lot and heads north along South Marginal Road to the East 55th Street Bridge, where it turns left (toward the lake), crosses Memorial Shoreway, and heads south along the lake front. You will pass the Gordon Shore Boat Club, the Forest City Yacht Basin, and the Lakeside Yacht Basin. In the distance you can see Cleveland's Municipal Stadium, home of the Browns and the Indians. You will also pass the Burke Lakefront Airport, the U.S. Coast Guard station, and the Donald Gray Gardens before reaching the stadium. On your way you will see a lot of regular Cleveland runners, called "Flats Rats," who run here in the flats daily. You can loop the stadium, about 440 yards around, and see a ball game after your run.

Running contacts:

Cleveland–West Road Runners Club sponsors Saturday morning fun runs below the Detroit Avenue bridge. The Cleveland–West RRC, P.O. Box 16243, Rocky River, Ohio 44116.

Ted Creighton, The Complete Runner, 2218 Lee Rd., Cleveland, Ohio 44101.

Dallas

Everybody runs in Big D, the home of Lt. Gen. R. L. Bohannon, M.D., president of the National Jogging Association, and Dr. Kenneth Cooper and his Aerobics Center.

Best runs: The Aerobics Activity Center at 12100 Preston Road has a track, marked in tenths of a mile, which explores a landscape of willows and crepe myrtle. Visitors must be accompanied by a member, and there is a small charge. The center is open Monday through Saturday, 5:30 a.m. to 9:30 p.m.; (214-233-3842).

Every day, at noon, joggers leave the downtown Dallas area for workouts. One favorite run starts at the Downtown YMCA at 12 p.m., and covers up to 8 miles along Turtle Creek Boulevard. You may run as much of that distance as you wish.

Weekends, runners favor the shores of White Rock Lake in Highland Park. Races and workouts usually begin in The Big Thicket, and the path, except for two miles, closely hugs the shoreline.

Running contacts:

The Downtown Branch YMCA is located at 605 North Ervay, Dallas, Texas 75201; (214-743-3251).

The Cross-Country Club of Dallas is at 6891 Avalon, Dallas, Texas 75214.

Denver

Talk about hills!

Denver rests on the eastern slopes of the Rocky Mountains. It's called "The Mile High City," and runners from closer-to-sea-level areas should get acclimated by being on the site for at least a week before starting out. Also, the sun can be stronger at this altitude, although city planners have planted Denver's parks with a variety of shade trees, a blessing to runner and stroller.

Best runs: Downtown Denver offers City Park along 17th Street between York and Colorado. The distance here is about 2.2 miles inside and 5 miles around the perimeter, mostly on grass. Or, try Washington Park at Downing and Virginia Streets, which has a 2.2-mile paved road dotted with drinking fountains. To the west, Sloans Lake includes a 2.9-mile sidewalk course.

Denver runners will gladly show a visitor some 46 miles of paths from the suburb of Littleton through Denver to Aurora, on the east side. This is the Highline Canal; in Littleton and Aurora the running clubs have kept the trail alongside the canal clear.

For hilly workouts, try the Arapahoe Loop. This 5-mile run in Littleton will challenge the best. Begin at Arapahoe High School (at University and Dry Creek Roads), head west to Broadway, south to County Line Road, and east. A turn at Mount County Line will bring you back to Arapahoe High School.

Running contacts:

Central Denver YMCA, 25 East 16th Ave., Denver, Colo. 80202; (303-861-8300).

The Denver Track Club, C/O Pat Conroy, 901 Kearney, Denver, Colo. 80220; (303-377-4718).

Rocky Mountain Road Runners, C/O Buzz Yancey, 129 Washington #5, Denver, Colo. 80203.

Gar Williams, former RRC national president, 6555 High Circle, Morrison, Colorado 80465.

Detroit

Home of the American motor car, Detroit is also a good place to use your legs to get around.

Best runs: Along the Detroit River, four miles from downtown, Belle Island offers three courses: the perimeter of 5.3 miles and AAU certified; a 5000-meter road course; a 1-mile loop. The courses are on pavement, with dirt paths running alongside.

Five miles north of downtown is Palmer Park with 4- and 5-mile courses. These paths are not well marked, however, and the runner might do well to run in Sherwood Forest, an elegant suburb, one block beyond.

In Chandler Park (at Edsel Ford Freeway, and Conner) a cinder path attracts joggers who run a figure-eight pattern with each loop counting 1.5 miles. Two miles north of downtown, Wayne State University has a 1.1-mile-per-lap track.

Running contacts:

The Belle Island Runners are 150 people who enjoy weekend jogs around the island, about 7 miles. Contact Dr. Edward Kozloff, 10144 Lincoln, Huntington Woods, Mich. 48070.

For indoor running try the YMCA Downtown Branch, 2020 Witherell St., Detroit, Mich. 48226; (314-WO 2-6126).

Hawaii

These islands have excellent temperatures and winds for running.

Best runs: There is lots of good running around Waikiki. The Ala Wai Canal is about 1.2 miles long. Near Mount Tantalus is a 10-mile loop, 5 miles up and 5 back, with great views of the Pacific. There is also a 1.7-mile loop around Kapiolani Park at the Kuhio end of Waikiki Beach, past the zoo. If you continue on, going up around Diamond Head crater, which includes the park, you'll cover 4.8 miles, with more long views of the ocean.

Kapiolani and Ala Moana Parks, cared for by the city, have running paths. You may want to start at the bandstand in Kapiolani and head out towards and over Diamond Head (following Kapiolani Blvd.-Diamond Head Rd.–Kahala Rd. to the golf course and back to the bandstand). That's 8 miles.

The Honolulu Marathon Clinic has maps with good running routes and miles marked on them. Contact Mimi Beams at the clinic, a member of the Greater New York Athletic Association who moved to Honolulu.

On the other islands—Maui, Kauai and Hawaii—you can run anywhere.

Running contacts:

Road Runners Club of Hawaii: Col. Thomas J. Ferguson (Ret.), 4191 Halvpa St., Honolulu, Hawaii 96818; or The Mid-Pacific Road Runners, C/O Gordon Dugan, 704 Ainapo St., Honolulu, Hawaii 96825.

Los Angeles

This is another runner's city. There are parks, and beaches along the Pacific Ocean, and lovely weather. The only drawback is the smog.

Best runs: Near downtown, Griffith Park offers hilly roads and 40 miles of bridle paths. Or, try the beach at Santa Monica, or the sidewalks overlooking Redondo Beach. San Vincente Boulevard, which offers a grassy stretch for 6 miles, is a favorite with LA joggers, who ignore warnings that the worst air pollution is found along highways.

This city also has excellent outdoor tracks. U.C.L.A., the University of California at Irvine, Long Beach State, Pierce College and Mt. San Antonio College have grass fields and good tracks. Santa Monica City College (near the beach) is a good meeting place for joggers of all ages.

One rule: Never jog on the freeways. Also, to avoid the worst smog hours, jog in the early morning or on weekends.

Running contacts:

The YMCAs are very active in Los Angeles, and two good ones are The Hollywood YMCA, 1553 N. Hudson Avenue, Hollywood, California, 90028; (213-467-4161). Or, West Side Family Branch, 11311 La Grange Ave., Los Angeles, California 90025 (213-477-1511).

Miami

Running in the summer is a trial here, but the other three seasons offer good weather.

Best runs: The bayside bike paths in Miami's Coconut Grove, the University of Miami campus and Miami-Dade Community College South. On Key Biscayne, the road from Crandon Park to Cape Florida Lighthouse (about 2.5 miles, some of it dirt) is a good run. Also, a bike path follows the contour of the beach for almost two miles. Birch State Park and Holiday Park in Fort Lauderdale offer good runs.

Running contacts:

The Road Runner's Club in Fort Lauderdale is very active, C/O Dennis Tunks, 731 Northeast 61st Street, Fort Lauderdale, Florida 33334.

The Downtown Branch YMCA, 40 Northeast Third Avenue, Miami, Florida 33132; (305-374-8487).

Minneapolis

Some runners call this city "Eugene, Oregon, East." It is full of men and women who run everywhere, and a lot of them are national-class runners like Gary Bjorklund, Ron Daws, Steve Hoag, and Dr. Alex Ratelle.

One reason there are so many runners is that the paths and parks of Minneapolis encourage people to run. For three seasons of the year, this is a superb place for runners. In winter, some of them head indoors to the Downtown YMCA or other tracks. Hardy Minnesota Vikings plunge ahead, however, even during blizzards.

The whole parkway system in this city offers excellent runs. The Minnehaha Parkway may be best, with pedestrian paths stretching from Minnehaha Falls to Lake Harriet; put them all together, and you could run more than a marathon here. Better still, streets pass over or under the paths.

Best run: By far the greatest attraction is the running paths that loop the three major lakes of Minneapolis: Calhoun (3.1 miles around on the path), Harriet (2.6 miles), and Lake of the Isles (2.7 miles).

If you are downtown, you follow Hennipen Avenue and take a right on Franklin Avenue (or some less busy street) about 1.2 miles to the lakes. Now you can chew off as much mileage as you wish. Once on the lakes, you can run 50 miles without crossing more than a few streets, and the scenery is magnificent. There are two paths, for pedestrians and bicycles. Start at one spot, loop all three lakes, and return to the same spot, and you will cover exactly 10 miles.

Running Contacts:

Downtown Branch YMCA, 30 South Ninth Street, Minneapolis, Minn. 55402 (612) 332-2431

Minnesota Distance Runners Association, P.O. Box 14064, University Station, Minn. 55414 (612) 927-5815

Steve Hoag   Running World, 3511 West 70th Street, Minneapolis, Minn. 55402 (612) 925-1411

Gary Bjorklund   Body 'n' Sole, 1312 Southeast Fourth Street, Minneapolis, Minn. 55402 (612) 331-5680

New Orleans
There are long, isolated runs available along Lake Pontchartrain, and short jogs in City Park. But most runs in this gracious southern city begin at or pass the Gernon Brown Gymnasium at Harrison and Marconi Avenues. Here, too, begins the famous Mardi Gras Marathon.

Best runs: From the flagpole in front of the Gernon Gym, jog along Marconi toward the lake, left on Robert E. Lee Boulevard, right a mile later to West End Boulevard (which becomes Lakeshore Drive). Here, you can run for 15 miles, or shorter distances, by watching the painted markers and turning back when you wish. Saturday mornings, this course is crowded with local runners.

In downtown New Orleans, try Audubon Park on St. Charles Street across from Tulane University. On River Drive, just beyond the zoo, an "S (3)" painted on the pavement starts a 3-mile course that borders the park. Or, take Riverside Drive between Audubon Park and the Mississippi River, and follow it to the levee along the river.

Running contacts:

The New Orleans Track Club, C/O George Green, Apt. 100 N, 300 Ridge Lake, New Orleans, Louisiana 70001.

New York City
Be prepared to run with the famous and beautiful: Robert Redford, Joey Heatherton, Jerry Stiller, Donna De Verona, Joseph Heller, Jackie Onassis, Paul Simon, Spencer Haywood all work out at one of the city's YMCAs or in Central Park. Dustin Hoffman trained for and filmed *Marathon Man* around the park's popular reservoir. Mohammed Ali likes to run there as well—"floating like a butterfly."

Best runs: There is an unbelievable assortment. On the East Side of Manhattan, walk or jog to the East River promenade, which begins just north of the Queensboro Bridge at 61st Street, and run along the river north to Carl Schurz Park, home of Gracie Mansion, the mayor's official residence. Twenty city blocks equal one mile.

If you are staying near Central Park, you have every kind of running challenge at your door. Weekends and holidays year round, and summer weekdays from 10 a.m. to 4 p.m., as well as certain summer evenings, the interior roadway of the park is closed to cars. Joggers can run the complete loop, of 6 miles, or shorter loops of 5 miles by taking the cut-off at 102nd Street, and 4 miles by taking both the 102nd & 72nd Street cutoffs.

The park's reservoir between 86th and 96th Streets offers two paths. The upper cinder oval that borders the reservoir itself is 1.5 miles. The lower, softer bridle path covers 1.6 miles. Between 5 and 7 p.m. the reservoir area is filled with talkative runners. It's a social affair, which centers around the 90th Street and Fifth Avenue entrance. Here, too, on Saturday mornings, you'll usually find me teaching a Road Runner's Club beginners class starting at 10 a.m. We generally have more than 200 beginner and intermediate runners out there ready to go.

Other runs in Central Park include the Oval, just above the pond by Belvedere Castle (a weather station) and Shakespeare-in-the-Park Theater at 82nd Street. Distances are marked on the pavement; a dirt path parallels the hard surface. In the evenings, the view of lighted Midtown Manhattan is unequalled.

Another Manhattan park with a good run is Riverside Park, on the upper West Side along the Hudson River. There is an outdoor 220-yard cinder track at West 72nd Street in the park, which is popular with runners like Arnold Spellun and author Kitty Lance. A longer run begins at 72nd Street and follows the upper promenade for 5 miles to the tower of Riverside Church, which you can see in the distance. One section of this run is marked each quarter mile by paint on the wide sidewalk.

On Wednesday evenings at 6:45, the Road Runner's Club and the Greater New York AA sponsor a group run that begins on West 63rd Street between Broadway and Central Park West. We usually meet under the YMCA's awning and jog over to Riverside Park at 72nd Street, and follow the Hudson to the George Washington Bridge. That's 13 miles. You can run with the group as far as you wish, but the run usually ends back on West 63rd, where everyone heads over to Martin's Bar for 45-cent draft beers.

Also from the West 63rd Street Y, head into Central Park and run on the cinder bridle path which joins the one at the reservoir, a distance of about 1.5 miles. Other Y's in Manhattan are just as well located. The Vanderbilt Y on East 47th Street is a short jog from the footpaths along the East River Drive. Like the West Side Y, the downtown McBurney Y on West 23rd Street has an indoor track, or you can run from the Y to the West Side Highway, which is closed to cars until a plan to rebuild is decided upon. From 23rd Street a 6-mile run along the highway would take you south to Battery Park and back. (Stop in to see McBurney member John Weiss at *Runner's World*, a nearby runner's store, for advice about shoes and running from a local marathoner.)

Other runs include the paths in Brooklyn's Prospect Park, a 5-mile cross-country trail in Van Cortlandt Park in the Bronx, Queen's Alley Pond Park, and Staten Island's Clove Lake Park. All are excellent running spots, although a bit far from midtown hotels.

Running contacts:

The New York Road Runner's Club hosts more than 100 races a year, including the nation's biggest marathon and women's race: the New York City Marathon in October; the 10 kilometer "Mini-Marathon" in late May or early June. Contact Fred Lebow, President, New York Road Runners, P.O. Box 881 FDR Station, New York, New York 10022; (212-595-3389).

The West Side YMCA has an indoor, padded track, 23 laps to the mile; 5 West 63rd Street, New York, New York 10023; (212-787-4400). The Vanderbilt Y is at 224 East 47th Street, New York, N.Y. 10017; (212-PL 5-2410). The McBurney Y, 215 West 23rd St., New York, N.Y. 10011; (212-CH 3-1982). The YM/YWHA also has an indoor track at 92nd Street and Lexington Avenue; (212-427-6000).

Philadelphia

In the movie *Rocky*, Sylvester Stallone jogs through this city and ends up sprinting up the steps of the Philadelphia Museum of Art at dawn. It's a poignant scene, and Philadelphia joggers recognized it also as almost impossible: The total run would have covered almost 30 miles.

Still, the best runs are found around the Schuylkill River (pronounced Sku-kill) or in Fairmount Park. One of the finest runs in Philadelphia follows the Schuylkill in Fairmount. A 5-mile course starts near Belmont Plateau; it is hilly and tough, and about 15 minutes from downtown. Near the Art Museum along the Schuylkill, follow the East River Drive. Joggers can run on either grass or pavement.

To follow some of Rocky's route, try The Parkway from Center City out toward Fairmount Park.

In downtown Philadelphia, an ideal all-weather track is the University of Pennsylvania's Tartan oval at Franklin Field. Take South Street to 34th to reach the field.

Running contacts:

Central Branch YMCA, 1421 Arch Street, Philadelphia, Pennsylvania 19102; (215-569-1400).

The Mid-Atlantic Road Runners Club, C/O Joe McLihinney, 908 Cottman Street, Philadelphia, Pennsylvania 19111; (215-342-7600).

Pittsburgh

Although Pittsburgh is a sprawling city, the visitor is seldom more than 10 minutes from a good run.

Best runs: Downtown, the Golden Triangle YMCA holds a daily run at noon. Route: From the YMCA to the Monongahela River Wharf to the confluence of the Monongahela and Allegheny Rivers, upriver along the Allegheny, down the east bank encircling Three Rivers Stadium, returning across the Fort Duquesne Bridge. The Y is close to the William Penn and Hilton Hotels. Call 412-261-5820 for that day's run.

There are also 36 parks in Pittsburgh with running paths. One run is in the North Hills around North Park Lake, exactly 5.1 miles. Joggers meet there most mornings. University of Pittsburgh joggers like the 10,000-meter bike trail in Schenley Park. The park is primitive, much as it was when the French and Indians fought there more than 250 years ago. There are also excellent trails in Frick Park near the outer edge of the city.

Running contacts:

Golden Triangle YMCA, 304 Wood Street, Pittsburgh, Pa. 15222.

The Greater Pittsburgh Road Runner's Club, C/O Stuart Levy, 818 MacArthur Drive, Pittsburgh, Pa. 15228; (412-341-4141). Or, the Allegheny Mountain RRC, C/O Shirley McDaniels, 721 Vallevista Avenue, Pittsburgh, Pa. 15234.

Portland/Eugene

Oregon has as many runners as raindrops—and it rains a lot there. Eugene, home of the late Steve Prefontaine, is the earth's center of jogging. The University of Oregon runners there fill pathways and roads, as do the Oregon State joggers at Corvallis.

Eugene claims the title "Jogging Capital of the World." The University of Oregon track meets are standing-room-only affairs filled with knowledgeable, enthusiastic spectators. Jim Ferris, men's coach of the Greater New York AA, and a former U. of O. trackman, claims that "the town explodes with runners" of all ages and abilities.

Best Eugene runs: The bike path along the canal; the Alton Baker 10,000-meter wood chip path called "Pre's Trail" after Prefontaine. There is also good running in Hendrix Park, and along the streets of Eugene, in Laurelwood golf course outside town, or at the U. of O. track, which is open 24 hours a day. For local information, check in at The Athletic Dept. at the Eugene Mall, where you'll find some of our top runners.

Portland offers some fine runs within easy reach of downtown. Best runs: Duniway Park, on the foot of the West Hills near SW Fifth Avenue. A bicycle path leads into the hills for about 3.4 miles; the grade is steep and a good workout. Bonus: the trail is paved, the route overgrown with ferns, trees, grass and bushes. The Willamette River winds below, and on clear days—a rare occasion—you can see Mt. Hood.

Mt. Tabor Park on the east side of Portland covers 200 acres on the site of an extinct volcano. Forest Park, a little farther out, is a 7000-acre preserve with some 30 miles of cross-country paths.

If you have a car, try Seaside over on the Pacific Ocean. There, the Trail's End marathon and a 7-mile beach run are held in February and August. Or, drive twelve miles northwest to Sauvie Island, where the Willamette flows into the Columbia River. This flat agricultural island and waterfowl flyway features a 12-mile loop road, the site in November of an annual Island Marathon.

Running contacts:

Portland YMCA, 831 SW Sixth St., Portland, Oregon 97204; (503-223-6161).

The Oregon Road Runners, with 500 members, is very active. Contact Ken Weidkamp, 14230 SW Derby Street, Beaverton, Oregon 97005.

St. Louis

If you are planning to meet anyone in St. Louie, Louie, be sure to pack your running shoes.

Best runs: Forest Park, near the Kingshighway hotels and across the street from the Chase Park-Plaza Hotel, offers the best paths. It is also within a jog of the St. Louis YMCA.

Forest Park is four miles west of downtown. The asphalt bicycle path loops in a 10-kilometer arch past fountains and lagoons, up steep hills, alongside playing fields and the St. Louis Zoo. A fork allows the runner to follow the J. F. Kennedy Forest route (6.53 kilometers) or stay outside (6.2).

In the suburbs, try the Tartan track at Florissant Valley Community College. Next to it is a 1.4-mile course with a steep hill. In University City, Heman Park has a 1.5-mile path. On the Illinois side of the Mississippi, the annual River Run in November features 10 miles of grey, misty views between Principia College in Elsah to the Alton city limits.

Running contacts:

The St. Louis YMCA Track Club runs a March marathon over the 1904 Olympic course, and includes a 10-kilometer race and a 1-mile fitness run. Contact the St. Louis YMCA Track Club, Downtown YMCA, 1528 Locust St., St. Louis, Missouri 63103; (314-GE 6-4100). The Y also has an indoor, banked oval track, 26 laps to the mile.

The Road Runner's Club may be reached through Jerry Kokesh, 1226 Orchard Village Drive, Manchester, Mo. 63011.

San Diego

The variety of San Diego is exciting: flat beaches, steep hillsides, rugged canyons, green parks and bayside marathon courses.

Best runs: Balboa Park is almost in the center of San Diego. Runners meet there to work out on either the grass or paved running paths. Another favorite route is Rosecrans Street to Cabrillo Monument Drive to the monument itself, which juts into the sky along the Pacific Ocean. This is a great sunset run. Or, try the beaches at Coronado; the crescent view is unsurpassed anywhere.

Workouts are also popular along the magnificent, steep, winding hills of La Jolla (pronounced La Hoy-ya) north of the city. Beyond La Jolla, a long beach stretches for 20 miles; runners may pass nude bathers, hang gliders and other California fauna. Hills and altitude training await the serious runner to the east of San Diego, where Penasquitoes Canyon contains a tough 22-mile marathon course. The Laguna Mountains, an hour's drive, reach 6,000 feet and offer unlimited paths and roads for mountain running.

Running contacts:

Bill and Donna Gookin are excellent long-distance runners. She teaches women runners; he invented the famous runner's drink, ERG. Contact them at the San Diego Track Club, 5946 Wenrich Drive, San Diego, California 92120.

Downtown YMCA, 1115 Eighth Avenue, San Diego, California 92101; (714-232-7451).

San Francisco

This city has more hills than Rome, and cable cars to climb them. But there are also flat places to run, if that's your preference, and for a unique run, the lovely Golden Gate Bridge.

Best runs: one of the best in the West begins with a cable car ride. From the major hotels, take the Hyde Street cable car, which passes the St. Francis Hotel and within a block of the Hilton, Mark Hopkins and Fairmount Hotels. At Hyde Street, where the cable car ends, run in either direction past outstanding restaurants, stores, maritime museums and fishing boats. This is the Embarcadero, filled with runners from the Y and downtown hotels. One hotel, the Hyatt-Union Square, offers its running guests free rides to and from the waterfront.

Or, for the best run, turn west to Marina Green Boulevard, and follow the lush grass toward the Presidio. By jogging through Crissy Field, you cover 2 miles and reach the Golden Gate Bridge, which you can run across on the fenced sidewalk (1.5 miles).

Or, from the same cable car stop, try the flat run to the Ferry Building 2 miles away. Continue to Third Street, and run by the dockyards toward Candlestick Park and the Cow Palace, 10 miles from the start.

There are also paths in Golden Gate Park, which is four miles by a half-mile wide, and reaches to the Pacific. A 5-mile AAU certified course circles Lake Merced near the ocean, south of Golden Gate Park.

For hill work, you've picked a good city. Try running from the Maritime Museum to California Street and return—up Nob Hill. (If you are staying at the Hopkins or Fairmount Hotel, you can run from your front door.) Or, run 1.5 miles to the Coit Tower. Twin Peaks, to the southwest, offers a steep mile with a sweeping view of city and harbor.

Running contacts:

The Dolphin-South End Running Club (DSE) is led by the barrel-chested, sixty-five-plus legendary Walter Stack. They run every Sunday morning, and turn out runners by the hundreds. Awards are made annually on a point system: one point for every mile of racing; one point for every 20 miles of training. The DSE, C/O Walt Stack, 321 Collingwood St., San Francisco, California 94114; (415-647-9459).

One of the largest running clubs on the West Coast is the West Valley Track Club. Contact Jack Leydig, P.O. Box 1551, San Mateo, California 94401.

Also, the Bay Area Road Runners Club, C/O Bill Flodberg, 12925 Foothill Ave., San Martin, California 95046; (408-683-2810).

Seattle

This city offers mountains, lakes, the sea and wonderful running companions.

Best runs: One includes Lake Washington Drive, which covers 3 miles between the original Floating Bridge and Seward Park. On clear days, Mt. Rainier and the Cascade Range are visible. To extend your run another 3 miles include Seward Park Peninsula by following the beach road. The path is paved, with dirt alongside.

Or, begin at the University of Washington on Union Bay, and follow two options: Either run south to the university's Arboretum, which includes several miles of dirt paths through woods and bird sanctuaries. Or, follow the Bert Gilman Trail, converted from an old railroad line, west along Lake Union. This trail follows the ship canal through park areas, fishing boat marinas and railroad tracks to Puget Sound—a distance of 3 miles.

At the locks, you might want to continue toward Ft. Lawton and Discovery Park, a route with running trails that follow high bluffs. One road descends to the beach and a mile of variety.

Green Lake, north of the University of Washington, may be Seattle's best known running spot. A paved path course 28 miles traces the lake's shore. There are rest rooms and a nearby zoo.

Running contacts:

The Pacific Northwest A.C., C/O Bill Roe, 2557 25th Avenue East, Seattle, Washington 98112; (206-325-3167). The Seattle Downtown YMCA has an indoor track at 909 Fourth Avenue, Seattle, Washington 98104; (206-MA 2-5208).

Washington, D.C.

This is a jogger's city. Runners line the major roadways and follow paths through their favorite parks every day. The only drawback is the fact that, in summer, Washington steams.

Best runs: Loop the Tidal Basin during cherry blossom time. This short run of about 1 mile starts at the Lincoln Memorial and follows the Ohio Drive to the D Street Bridge, and return. To lengthen the run, lap the basin and follow Ohio Drive into East Potomac Park to Hains Point. A loop around the park, with splendid views of the Potomac, is about 3 miles.

The most famous run follows the old C & O Canal. Joggers may enter the towpath at 34th Street NW, just below M Street in Georgetown. The path follows the canal for about 5 miles; on its left side (leaving Washington) are mile markers. Horse-drawn passenger barges make daily trips along the canal in summer.

Washington has more than 47 miles of bike paths, and some of these offer good and safe running, too. From a downtown hotel, Rock Creek Park may be reached by public transportation (or a short run). Or, hill work may be preferred along Embassy Row on Massachusetts Avenue. Follow Massachusetts to Westmoreland Circle, about 3.5 miles and up some tough hills.

During winter or after dark (when the parks are unsafe), runners can try the Central YMCA, with its banked, rubberized track (25 laps to the mile). This Y also hosts the annual Cherry Blossom Classic, a 10-mile run that coincides with the Cherry Blossom Festival every April. More than 3,000 runners show up. A fitness run is held at the same time.

Running contacts:

Jeff Darman, National President, RRC of America, 2737 Devonshire Place NW, Washington, D.C. 20008.

The DC Road Runners, C/O Ray Morrison, 120 Eastmoor Drive, Silver Spring, Maryland 20910.

The Central YMCA, 1736 G Street NW, Washington, D.C. 20006; (202-626-8250).

Where to run (abroad)

Traveling overseas? Foreigners are getting used to Americans jogging along their quiet, lovely streets in shorts and bright running shoes. Better yet, Americans are earning an international reputation as long-distance runners. Whatever your distance, be sure to pack a few extra club or U.S.A. running shirts to trade.

London

A charming and leafy town to run in, although the British may still be a little surprised by Americans jogging about.

An easy, delightful run encircles Hyde Park–Kensington Gardens. Start at the main gate to Hyde Park (Hyde Park Corner), at Knightsbridge and Park Lane. You may either run up Park Lane to Bayswater Road (use the sidewalk), or enter the park on one of the paths along Rotten Row, a former sand track for horses. Either way, take the cut-off that connects Bayswater with Kensington Road and crosses the Serpentine (1 mile). Circling the entire park would cover about 3 miles, passing the London Museum and the Albert Memorial.

From almost any hotel in central London, an easy jog puts you along the Thames River. The promenade along Victoria Embankment offers a grand view of the Houses of Parliament, Waterloo Bridge, and (if you've the stamina) by running along Upper and Lower Thames Street, Tower Bridge and the Tower of London. You jog by the gate where Elizabeth I was led to imprisonment. From Westminster to Tower Bridge is about 2.5 miles. The best run would be along Victoria Embankment from Westminster to Blackfriars Bridge, about 1.2 miles.

Green Park is worth a loop or two, as is Saint James Park, with its ducks and enormous pelicans, and elegantly dressed Queen's guards marching to and from Buckingham Palace. The two parks connect, and a loop of them both would cover about 2.5 miles.

Montreal

One of the elegant cities of North America. Its excellent restaurants will help you restore glycogens at a very modest cost. Most midtown hotels are on major streets, and running in a park requires a ride on the Metro, the best subway system on the North American continent.

Parc Mont-Royal, with its observatory and lake (Lac des Castors), offers several good runs along park paths. Start at the observatory and take the path to the left (south). At the first major fork, you may swing right and make a 2-mile loop back to the observatory by passing along Voie Camillien-Houde or by running left and continuing in a long loop to the lake and back (about 4 miles). The park contains good hills for runners seeking that training.

Another run, reached by Metro, is on Île Sainte-Hélène. This island, site of Expo '67 and the Man and His World exhibit, contains a short (1.5 mile) inner sidewalk loop, and a magnificent 2.5-mile run along the St. Lawrence, part of it facing the city. There are restrooms and drinking fountains, and an amusement park for the kids.

Near the site of the Olympic Village are a golf course, park, and botanical garden. Run and reminisce about the games of 1976. Check with the YMHA or YMCA for the Olympic marathon course, and retrace the steps of Shorter and Cierpinski.

On weekends or evenings when traffic is lighter, you might run from your hotel to Old Montreal, the site of the original settlement 300 years ago. Place d'Armes is a landmark on the way, with Nôtre Dame church. The area is filled with restaurants, boutiques, antique shops.

Nairobi (Kenya)
A perfect city to run in, located in East Africa. Kenya has turned out several world-class runners, such as Mike Boit, Kipchoge Keino, Henry Rono, Wilson Waigwa. You may even be applauded in your U.S.A. running shirt.

The city is 5,500 feet above sea level on the vast, game-filled Athi Plain. It is modern, pleasant, cool—daytime temperatures rarely exceed 80 degrees Fahrenheit, although it is only 87 miles from the equator.

Nairobi is compact. From the central hotels (New Stanley, Hilton, Inter-Continental), the runner may try a 1.5-mile rectangle along Sergeant Ellis Avenue toward the Parliament buildings to Uhuru Highway to Harambee Avenue to Government Road.

You may also follow the students footpath around Uhuru Park, across from the Parliament buildings and close to the Inter-Continental. Near the Norfolk Hotel, Nairobi University sports grounds on Uhuru Highway feature a quarter-mile track and running paths. After your runs on the sports grounds, jog up to the traffic circle (called a roundabout), turn right up Ainsworth Hill, and then right again to the Nairobi Snake Park. Here you will find (in glass cages) 200 varieties of snakes, most of them highly poisonous, like the green and black mambas, cobras, and the ugly Gabon viper. Viewing them will give you excellent knee lift next time you run in the African grass.

The best run in Nairobi may be at the Muthaiga Country Club, which has a manicured golf course free of lions. If you can get someone to invite you over, an early morning (pre-golf) run on the course is beautiful.

Swahili is the *lingua franca* of East Africa. A friendly wave and "*Habari*" or "*Hujambo*" (but never both) will elicit smiles and greetings. Avoid hotel Swahili like "*jambo*"; that labels you as a tourist.

Paris

This may still be the world's most beautiful city. The best way to enjoy it is to move around a lot. Walking before you run may be a wise first step, to plan your path. You might even try a tour bus to get oriented.

Once you know your way around, you'll want to try several runs. Lance Wyman, of Wyman & Cannon in New York, started running in Central Park, and during a business trip, put in 4 miles along the Seine and sent ecstatic postcards back to envious American friends.

One route, part of Wyman's path, starts at the Louvre at the foot of the Champs Elysées, near the Seine, to the Palais de Chaillot, across the river from the Eiffel Tower. There cross the Seine, run along rue de L'Université to the bridge at the Louvre, and return. This route passes architecture that ranges from medieval to nineteenth century. If you wish to run along the river, go down the steps to the path. This will mean, however, that you will have to climb stairs and cross streets at some bridges. The run covers about 8 miles. It can be extended by continuing to the Île de la Cité, the island in the middle of the Seine, site of Notre-Dame Cathedral.

Or, you may want to run around the Place de la Concorde (which is dangerous to cross because of motor traffic) to the rue de Rivoli. Cross at the lights and proceed past the American Embassy to the elegant gardens of the Champs Elysées. Run slightly uphill to the Arc de Triomphe (about 2 miles).

There are other runs: to the Latin Quarter, Montmartre, and in the Bois de Boulogne. A little French is necessary, plus some francs and the address of your hotel in case you tire or get lost.

Sydney, Australia

This is one of the best cities to run in on the Australian continent. Tourists will find the native runners friendly, helpful in pointing out running paths, and very good.

There are three outstanding runs in this city.

The most obvious is Centennial Park, the central park of Sydney, off Oxford Street behind the historical area of Paddington. There you will discover lovely homes with cast-iron balconies like those in New Orleans. The park is huge, almost 400 acres, with running paths and good shade.

Another excellent running area includes the bays behind King's Cross, the Times Square of Sydney. The bays, by contrast, are quaint with wide sidewalks. Sydney is a large city with inlets like fingers probing into it. These form a series of little bays pointing eastward from the city. The sidewalks connect them, and the runs are superb. One can go from Elizabeth Bay to Rushcutter's, Double Bay, and Rose Bay, each with its own park and sidewalks. The only hazard comes at night, when some of the wild life from King's Cross spills into the area.

Finally, try Bondi Beach, the most famous spot in Sydney. There is a wide sidewalk here, too, and one can run all the way to Tamarama Beach, about two miles, along a lovely uphill and downhill course.

The big running event in Sydney is the annual City-to-Surf race held in August. It is similar in theme and crowd to the Bay-to-Breakers run in San Francisco. The starting line is at Martin Place near the main post office in downtown Sydney, and the route climbs uphill for much of its 7 miles. But the glory comes when the 7,000 to 10,000 runners finish at the beach. They just keep running into the water.

Toronto

A lovely Canadian city with trees and flowers, new malls, and a charming mixture of old architecture and modern buildings. There are parks with water fountains or vendors for buying drinks. Marcy Schwam, a marathon runner who has covered Toronto, calls it "gorgeous."

One of the best runs begins in High Park with its difficult winding trails. Start at the corner of Bloor Street and Lakeshore Boulevard, and run during the daytime when you can see everything. Lakeshore has a wide sidewalk that runs for miles and passes a bread factory with delicious odors.

Try Queens Park. The Ontario Parliament buildings form part of this park, which is oval-shaped and very scenic. The oval forms a half-mile loop.

Or jog over to Sunnybrook Park at Leslie and Eglinton streets. Here is where the serious runners shape up. From the top of the park to the bottom and back they run a full 12 miles. This popular park is traffic-free, and you can adjust the distance run to your training level.

Tip: Anyone visiting Toronto is invited to drop by the YMCA (416 921-5171) and talk to the local runners. The Y also has maps of the different running courses and race routes in the Toronto area. They're a good bunch of runners.

Also, visit the CN Tower, the largest free-standing structure in the world. If plain running isn't enough of a thrill, the elevators on the outside of the building are glass-walled, and your descent is like a free fall out of the sky.

Highlights of Your
Running Travels

Races/Racing contacts

JANUARY

Orange Bowl Marathon
Miami, Fla.

Jose Rodriguez
7653 NW 74th Avenue
Tamarac, Fla. 33319

Mission Bay Marathon
San Diego, Calif.

Marathon
2691 Palace Drive
San Diego, Calif. 92123

Mardi Gras Marathon
New Orleans, La.

NOTC
Box 30491
New Orleans, La. 70190

FEBRUARY

Trails End Marathon
Seaside, Ore.

Chamber of Commerce
Box 7
Seaside, Ore. 97138

Carolina Marathon
Columbia, S.C.

Jim LaBonte
2600 Bull Street
Columbia, S.C. 29205

Gasparilla Classic, 15 kilometers
Tampa, Fla.

Gasparilla Distance Classic
City Hall
Tampa, Fla. 33602

MARCH

Bankathon, 30 kilometers

Burke Adams
21 Chestnut Court
Rensselaer, N.Y. 12144

International Women's Marathon
Atlanta, Ga.

Katherin Switzer
Avon Products, Inc.
9 West 57th Street
New York, N.Y. 10019

Tucson Sun Run, 15 kilometers
Tucson, Ariz.

Kai Haber, M.D.
2520 Carnivo La Zorrela
Tucson, Ariz. 85718

APRIL

Cherry Blossom Classic
10 and 2 miles
Washington, D.C.

Jeff Darman
2737 Devonshire Place NW
Washington, D.C. 20008

Boston Marathon
Boston, Mass.
(Race requires sub-3:00:00 men;
   sub-3:30:00 men over 40 and women.)

Will Cloney
Boston AA
150 Causeway St.
Boston, Mass. 02114

Jacksonville River Run, 15 kilometers
Jacksonville, Fla.

Jacksonville Track Club
P.O. Box 515
Jacksonville, Fla. 32201

MAY

Bay-to-Breakers, 7.6 miles
San Francisco, Calif.

Frank Geis
PA-AAU Office
942 Market Street, No. 201
San Francisco, Calif. 94102

National Capital Marathon
Ottawa, Canada

Recreation
111 Sussex Drive
Ottawa, Canada KIN 5A 1

Indy Mini Marathon 13, 7 miles
Indianapolis, Ind.

Tom Bohlsen
Fellowship of Christian Athletes
333 North Pennsylvania Street, Suite
   934
Indianapolis, Ind. 46204

JUNE

New York City Women's
Mini-Marathon, 10 kilometers

New York Road Runners Club
P.O. Box 881, FDR Station
New York, N.Y. 10022

Garden of the Gods, 10 miles
Colorado Springs, Colo.

Rocky Mountain Road Runners
Buzz Yancey
129 Washington #5
Denver, Colo. 80203

Cascade Run Off, 15 kilometers
Portland, Ore.

Cascade Run Off
3500 First National Bank Tower
Portland, Ore. 97201

Westchester Half-Marathon
Westchester, N.Y.

New York Road Runners Club
P.O. Box 881, FDR Station
New York, N.Y. 10022

Sound-to-Narrows Run, 7.9 miles
Tacoma, Wash.

Pierce County Parks
2401 South 35th Street
Tacoma, Wash. 98409

JULY

Peachtree Road Run, 10 kilometers
Atlanta, Ga.

Bill Neece
2643 Laurel Ridge Drive
Decatur, Ga. 30033

San Francisco Marathon

Jim Scarnell
365 24th Avenue, No. 24
San Francisco, Calif. 94121

AUGUST

Falmouth Road Race, 7.1 miles
Falmouth, Mass.

John Carrol
Falmouth Recreation Dept.
Main Street
Falmouth, Mass. 02540

Pike's Peak Marathon, 14 miles up, 28
    miles round trip
Colorado Springs, Colo.

Merv Bennett
Pike's Peak YMCA
207 N. Nevada
P.O. Box 1694
Colorado Springs, Colo. 80901

SEPTEMBER

Charleston, W. Va., 15 miles

Dr. Donald Cohen
P.O. Box 1524
Charleston, W. Va. 25325

Virginia Ten Miler
Lynchburg, Va.

Rudy Straub
P.O. Box 1280
Lynchburg, Va. 24505

Mayor Daley Marathon
Chicago, Ill.

Ruth Ratney
900 N. Michigan Avenue
Chicago, Ill. 60611

OCTOBER

New York City Marathon

New York Road Runners Club
P.O. Box 881, FDR Station
New York, N.Y. 10022

Skylon Marathon
Buffalo, N.Y., to Niagara Falls, Canada

Frank Neal
10 Beard Avenue
Buffalo, N.Y. 14214

Labatt's Freedom Trail Road Race,
    8 miles
Boston, Mass.

Labatt's Freedom Trail Road Race
P.O. Box 84
Somerville, Mass. 02143

NOVEMBER

Marine Corps Reserve Marathon
Washington, D.C.

Marine Corps RESP
Washington, D.C. 20380

Road Runners Club of America
  National Age Group
  Cross-Country Championship

Barry Geisler
New York Road Runners Club
P.O. Box 881, FDR Station
New York, N.Y. 10022

DECEMBER

Honolulu Marathon

Marathon Association
Box 27244
Chinatown, Honolulu, Hawaii 96827

Fiesta Bowl Marathon
Scottsdale, Ariz.

Fiesta Bowl
3410 East Van Buren
Phoenix, Ariz. 85008

Running publications

Footnotes
Road Runner's Club of America
1584 Spruce Drive
Kalamazoo, Mich. 49008 (Free to members)

The Jogger
National Jogging Association
919 18th Street N.W., Suite 830
Washington, D.C. 20006 ($15 membership fee; appears 10 times a year)

The Marathoner
Box 366
Mountain View, Calif. 94042 ($10 a year; appears quarterly)

New York Running News
Box 881, FDR Station
New York, N.Y. 10022 ($10 includes Road Runners Club membership)

Running Times
12808 Occoquan Road
Woodbridge, Va. 22192 ($10 a year; appears monthly)

The Runner
One Park Avenue
New York, N.Y. 10017 ($12 a year charter subscription; appears monthly)

Running
Box 350
Salem, Ore. 97308 ($5 a year; appears quarterly)

Runner's Gazette
102 W. Water Street
Lansford, Pa. 18232 ($6 for 12 issues; appears quarterly)

Running Review
645 S. Prince Street
Lancaster, Pa. 17603 ($9 a year; appears monthly)

Runner's World
Box 2680
Boulder, Colo. 80302 ($9.50 a year; appears monthly)

Yankee Runner
P.O. Box 237
Merrimac, Mass. 01860 ($5 for 18 issues a year)

Running/Fitness contacts

American Alliance for Health, Physical Education and Recreation
   (AAHPER)
1201 16th Street N.W.
Washington, D.C. 20037

American Association for Fitness in Business and Industry
C/O W. Brent Arnold, Fitness Director
Xerox Corporation
P.O. Box 2000
Leesburg, Va. 22075

American Heart Association
7320 Greenville Avenue
Dallas, Texas 75231

American Medical Joggers Association
Box 4704
North Hollywood, Calif. 91607

American Podiatry Association
20 Chevy Chase Circle N.W.
Washington, D.C. 20015

AAU
3400 West 86th Street
Indianapolis, Ind. 46268

National Jogging Association
c/o Gary K. Olson, Executive Director
919 18th Street N.W., Suite 830
Washington, D.C. 20006

National YMCA
c/o Clayton Myers, Ph.D.,
   Director, Cardio-vascular Health Program
291 Broadway
New York, N.Y. 10007

President's Council on Physical Fitness and Sports
400 Sixth Street S.W., Suite 3030
Washington, D.C. 20201

Road Runner's Club of America
c/o Jeff Darman, President
2737 Devonshire Place, N.W.
Washington, D.C. 20008

Walking

Walk before you jog, jog before you run. Mix walking with jogging and gradually shift the proportions in favor of jogging as the weeks go by. Walking stretches your muscles and helps condition them.

Older people or those who cannot run because of injury may walk briskly for 20 to 60 minutes.

Dr. Ron Lawrence, president of the American Medical Joggers Association, likes to have older people walk instead of jog since it is less stressful. He suggests that older people work up to walking 10 miles without discomfort before taking their first jogging step.

Monthly Summary

(Additional information and personal comments)

January

February

March

April

May

June

July

August

September

October

November

December

Notes